ATKINS DIET
FOR BEGINNERS

*100 HEALTHY AND EFFECTIVE ATKINS DIET
RECIPES FOR WEIGHT LOSS.
A BEGINNER'S GUIDE TO START FEELING GREAT*

© Copyright 2021 - All rights reserved.

The content contained within this book may not be reproduced, duplicated or transmitted without direct written permission from the author or the publisher. Under no circumstances will any blame or legal responsibility be held against the publisher, or author, for any damages, reparation, or monetary loss due to the information contained within this book. Either directly or indirectly.

Legal Notice:

This book is copyright protected. This book is only for personal use. You cannot amend, distribute, sell, use, quote or paraphrase any part, or the content within this book, without the consent of the author or publisher.

Disclaimer Notice:

Please note the information contained within this document is for educational and entertainment purposes only. All effort has been executed to present accurate, up to date, and reliable, complete information. No warranties of any kind are declared or implied. Readers acknowledge that the author is not engaging in the rendering of legal, financial, medical or professional advice. The content within this book has been derived from various sources. Please consult a licensed professional before attempting any techniques outlined in this book.

By reading this document, the reader agrees that under no circumstances is the author responsible for any losses, direct or indirect, which are incurred as a result of the use of information contained within this document, including, but not limited to, errors, omissions, or inaccuracies.

Table of Contents

INTRODUCTION 8
    WHAT IS THE ATKINS DIET? 8
    THE SCIENCE BEHIND ATKINS: HOW IT WORKS 9
    BENEFITS OF THE ATKINS DIET 9

CHAPTER 1: BREAKFAST 12
    1. Breakfast Stuffed Pepper, Mexican Style 13
    2. Arugula, Pear and Hazelnut Salad 14
    3. Asian Roll-ups with Chicken and Peanut Sauce 15
    4. Baked Egg and Asparagus 16
    5. Breakfast Tacos 17
    6. Breakfast Burger 18
    7. Salmon and Egg Stuffed Avocados 19
    8. Cream Cheese Pancakes 20
    9. Bacon, Egg & Cheese Casserole 21
    10. Vanilla and Marshmallow Smoothie 22
    11. Broccoli Egg Muffins 23
    12. Raspberry Bread 24
    13. Ham and Cheddar Omelet 25
    14. Mini Pancake Donuts 26
    15. Pizza Waffles 27
    16. Pancakes, Berries, Whipped Cream Breakfast 28
    17. Eggs and Healthy Vegetables Fried in Coconut Oil 29
    18. Protein Pancakes 30
    19. Almond and Coconut Mug Muffin 31

CHAPTER 2: SNACKS, SIDES, AND APPETIZERS 32
    1. Caesar Salad Dressing 33
    2. Peanut Coleslaw 34
    3. Pecan and Gorgonzola Salad 35
    4. Pepper Ranch Salad Dressing 36
    5. Oven-Baked Carrot Fries 37
    6. Zesty Baked Fries 38
    7. Cauliflower Mushroom Risotto 39
    8. Coconut Orange Creamsicle Fat Bombs 40
    9. Corndog Muffins 41
    10. Layered Fried Queso Blanco 42

11.	Pineapple Slaw	43
12.	Yummilicious Ginger Flan	44
13.	Atkins Coffee Eggnog	45
14.	Beet-Pickled Deviled Eggs	46
15.	Cashew Bread	47

CHAPTER 3: LUNCH 48

1.	Fish Strips, Basil & Feta Salad	48
2.	Salmon & Bok Choy	49
3.	Fish Fillet with Capers & Tomatoes	50
4.	Shrimp Scampi	51
5.	Chicken with Peanut Sauce	52
6.	Chicken with Onion & Fennel	53
7.	Rosemary Chicken	54
8.	Moroccan Beef Lettuce Wraps	55
9.	Steak Fajitas	56
10.	Beef and Eggplant	57
11.	Barbecue Pulled Beef	58
12.	Pumpkin Soup with Coconut and Curry	59
13.	Quick Seafood Chowder	60
14.	Atkins Diet Soup	61
15.	Blue Cheese and Bacon Soup	62
16.	Versatile Vegetable Soup	63
17.	Chili With Beef	64
18.	Low Carb Chicken	65
19.	Chicken Drumsticks	66
20.	Chicken Curry	67
21.	Green Curry Shrimp and Vegetables	68
22.	Mussels Veracruz	69
23.	Italian Sausage and Mussels	70
24.	Breaded Fish with Mustard & Basil Sauce	71
25.	Trout and Fennel Parcels	72

CHAPTER 4: DINNER 74

1.	Salmon Panatela	75
2.	Blackened Fish Tacos with Slaw	76
3.	Red Cabbage Tilapia Taco Bowl	77
4.	Sicilian-Style Zoodle Spaghetti	78
5.	Sour Cream Salmon with Parmesan	79
6.	Roasted Tomato and Chicken Pasta	80
7.	Oat Risotto with Mushrooms, Kale, and Chicken	81

8. Turkey and Tomato Sauce 82
9. Tomato Chicken and Chickpeas 83
10. Turkey with Leeks and Radishes 84
11. Low-Carb Pork Medallions 85
12. Easy Mozzarella & Pesto Chicken Casserole 86
13. Easy Taco Casserole Recipe 87
14. Parmesan Chicken Tenders 88
15. Broccoli & Cheddar Keto Bread Recipe 89
16. Bacon-Wrapped Chicken Tenders with Ranch Dip 90
17. Farmhouse Beans & Sausage 91
18. Chicken Al Forno & Vodka Sauce with Two Cheeses 92
19. Coconut Turkey 93
20. Hot Chicken and Zucchinis 94
21. Chicken Bacon Ranch Casserole 95
22. Sushi Shrimp Rolls 96
23. Grilled Shrimp with Chimichurri Sauce 97
24. Coconut Crab Patties 98
25. Shrimp in Curry Sauce 99
26. Tilapia with Olives & Tomato Sauce 100

CHAPTER 5: DESSERTS 102

1. Berries With Chocolate Ganache 102
2. Caramelized Pear Custard 104
3. Chocolate Brownie Drops 105
4. Baked Pear Fans 106
5. Chocolate Frosty 107
6. Ginger Flan 108
7. Vegan Atkins Carrot Cake Bites 109
8. Antipasto Skewers 110
9. Chocolate Avocado Ice Cream 111
10. Mocha Mousse 112
11. Strawberry Rhubarb Custard 113
12. Energy Bites with Turmeric 114
13. Ginger and Turmeric Smoothie 115
14. Coffee Cacao Protein Bars 116
15. Mango Cream Pie 117

CONCLUSION 119

Introduction

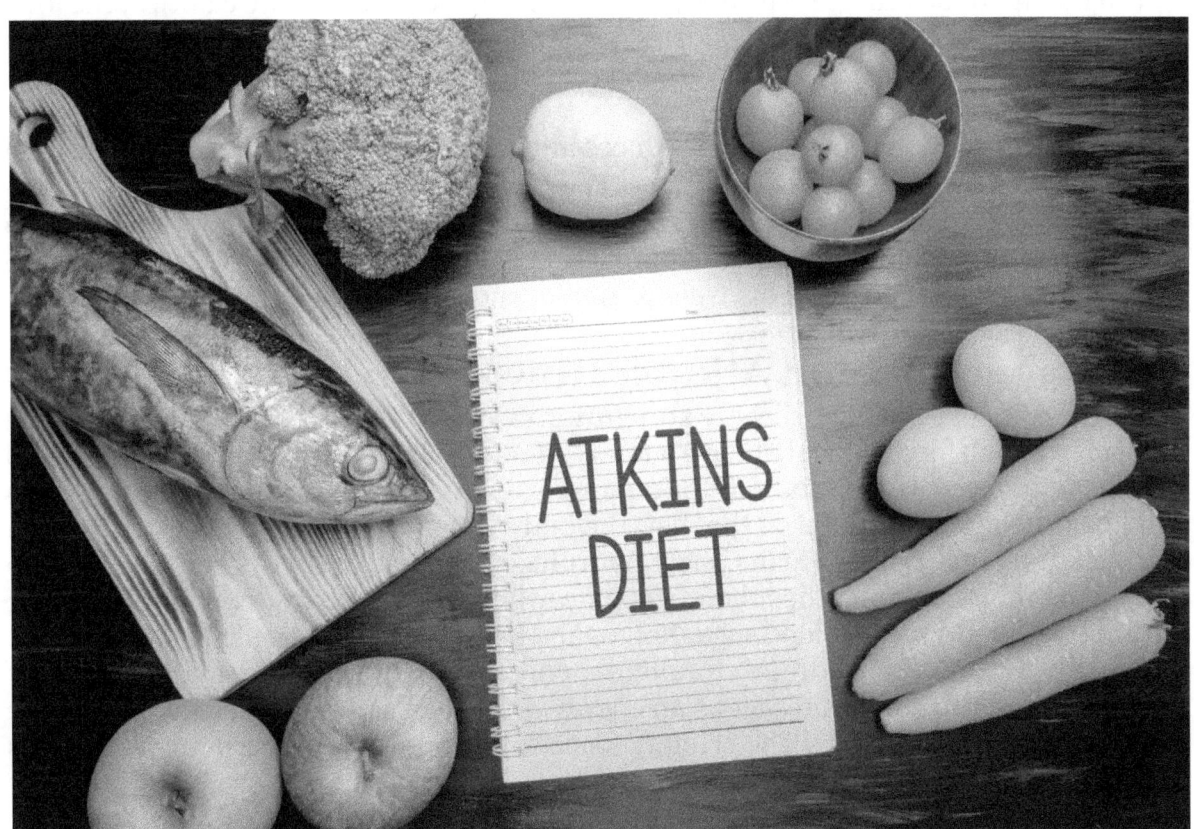

What Is the Atkins Diet?

The Atkins diet is one of the most successful commercial weight loss plans. It is named after Robert Atkins. This diet plan includes four phases and is similar to the low carbohydrate South Beach diet and the Low-GI diet plan. The focus of the Atkins diet is to consume a high protein, high fat, and low carbohydrate plan of eating. The diet promises to help you lose weight, as long as you are consuming a few carbohydrates and much protein and fat.

When following the Atkins diet plan, dieters restrict themselves to meals that are low on the Glycemic Index (GI). Foods having a low GI take some time for the stomach to digest and do not lead to an increase in blood sugar.

This successful diet plan was first introduced in the 1970s by Dr. Atkins. At that time, Dr. Atkins promoted this diet plan as much as possible and faced tremendous criticism and rejection. He went against the medical practices of the time. He introduced the Atkins diet plan in 1972. At that time, it was not the first low-carbohydrate diet plan but surely was the most successful one.

Dr. Atkins, based on his scientific research, said that a low-carbohydrate diet gives the body a metabolic advantage. The body, when burning fat, needs some calories; the low-carbohydrate diet expends those calories. Dr. Atkins suggested consuming 950 calories per day. The study created a huge backlash that there is no metabolic advantage, as you are just eating fewer calories per day.

According to Dr. Atkins, low-GI food reduces hunger as time is needed to digest the food. In 2002, a book was launched, known as "The New Diet Revolution." This book argues that the reason many low-carbohydrate diets fail is hunger. But in 2003, proving the idea wrong, the Atkin Nutritional Approach again gained popularity, as one of the Atkins diet followers stressed his weight loss journey, leading to a huge decline in the sale of food rich in carbohydrates.

The Science behind Atkins: How It Works

The mechanics of the Atkins diet are straightforward. You start to lose weight when you indulge in eating food items that have a low GI. Foods rich in fat, protein, and fiber help your body to feel satisfied and full for a more extended period of time. If lean protein and healthy fat are taken out of the diet, the body will always be in a food-deprivation mode. Indulging in eating organic, healthy fruits, lean meat, and nuts help the body to lose fat, as the Atkins diet flips the metabolic switch from carbohydrate burning to fat burning. This reduces the blood sugar spikes and helps diabetic patients in the long run. The body burns carbohydrates to obtain energy; when there is a deficiency of carbohydrates, the body stores fat as an energy source. When the fat starts to burn, the person begins to lose weight. The primary focus of the diet is on low carbohydrate meals that affect the body-boosting ability to burn more stored fat.

The massive reduction in sugar is the primary cause of weight loss in the Atkins diet plan.

We all know that the human body runs on glucose. When glucose is not available, fat, and then protein is used as a backup fuel source to the body.

Benefits of the Atkins Diet

- Helps the follower to lose weight in a limited time.
- Helps the follower to improve the HDL cholesterol.
- Claims to lower hypertension and control diabetes.
- Helps the follower to get rid of sugar cravings and food deprivation feeling by eating healthy food items.
- Helps the follower to get rid of stress and anxiety and improve brain health.
- Gives the follower better health and stamina.

- Increases energy.
- A low-carbohydrate diet, like the Atkins diet, helps to treat acne and gives glowing skin and stronger hair.
- Helps decrease heart disease risk factor.
- Helps alleviate heartburn and acid reflux.
- Reduces the symptoms of migraines and other headaches.
- Improves and helps reduce metabolic syndromes and cardiovascular diseases.

Since the Atkins diet was first introduced, it has changed over the past few years. Under the original plan, allowing everyone to eat eggs and bacon sounded appealing. The recent rules related to the Atkins diet have been modified extensively. The diet restricts more carbohydrates at the beginning and then allows flexibility afterward. No doubt, the Atkins diet gives promising results; it is an excellent way to lose weight and improve your health overall.

When following the Atkins diet, you get used to eating low carbohydrate food items. The diet does not allow refined sugar, such as white bread, pasta, or rice. The diet also helps teach you which carbohydrates are good for you and which are not.

Even if you have decided not to follow a diet, you will feel that healthy eating habits have developed and you will carry that knowledge forever. The Atkins diet plan does not stress the need to count calories. And keeping track of calories is quite a frustrating process. The calories are just one aspect of losing weight.

If you love eating meat and can't exclude it from your diet, and still want to lose weight, then be happy. The Atkins diet is all about the pleasure of eating the most delicious foods, like steaks, fried chicken, and burgers.

CHAPTER 1:

Breakfast

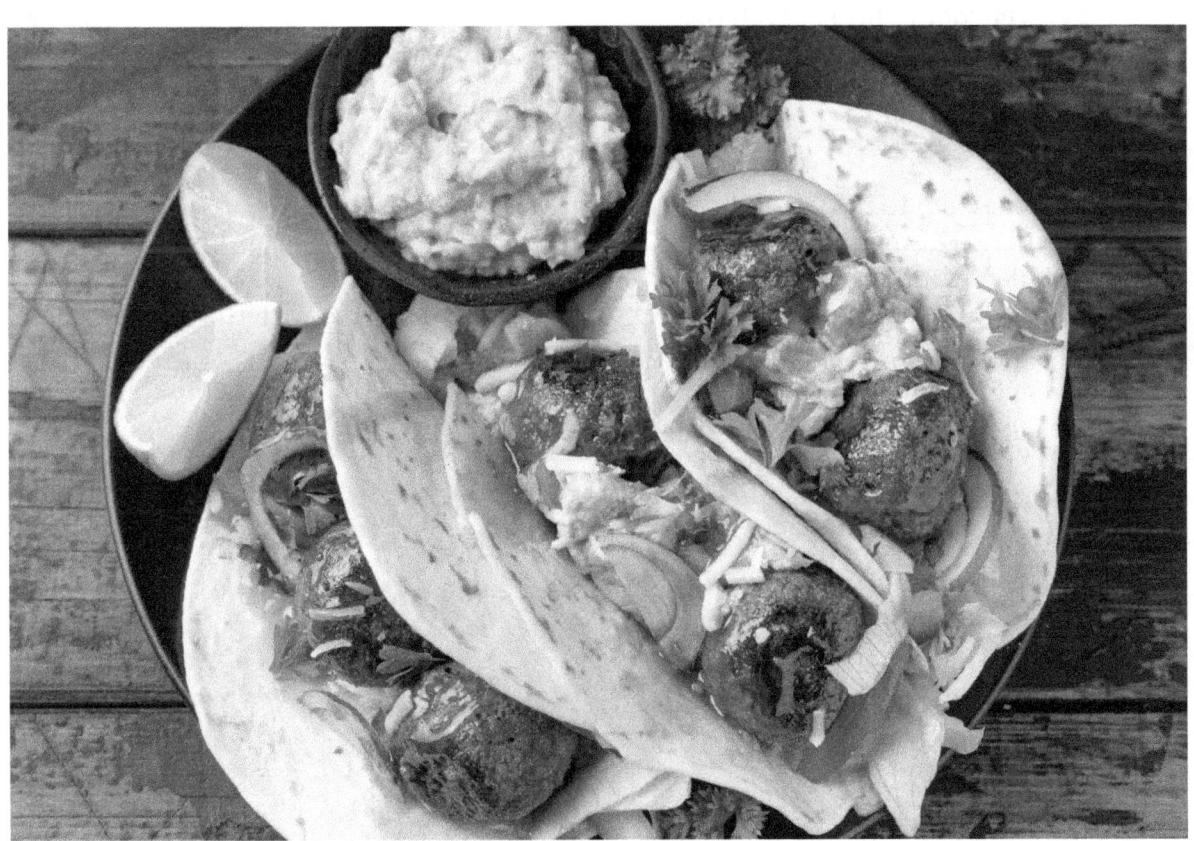

1. Breakfast Stuffed Pepper, Mexican Style

Preparation Time: 5 minutes
Cooking Time: 25–30 minutes
Servings: 1
Ingredients:

- 1 oz. pork and beef chorizo
- 1 oz. 80% lean ground beef
- 2 tablespoons chopped onion
- ¼ oz cheddar cheese, grated
- 1 large egg, beaten
- 1 medium sweet red peppers, cut in half lengthwise, seeds and white ribs removed

Directions:

1. Preheat oven to 400°F and line a baking sheet with foil.
2. In a pan over medium heat, cook chorizo and ground beef, crumbling meat while it cooks. Drain off excess fat.
3. Place cooked meat mixture in a mixing bowl and combine with the onion, cheese, and egg.
4. Fill pepper half with the meat mixture and place on the prepared baking sheet. Bake for 25–30 minutes and serve hot.

Nutrition:

- **Calories:** 326
- **Fat:** 24 g
- **Net Carbs:** 5 g
- **Protein:** 21 g

2. Arugula, Pear and Hazelnut Salad

Preparation Time: 5 minutes
Cooking Time: 10 minutes
Servings: 4
Ingredients:
- 10 oz. arugula
- ½ cup gorgonzola cheese, crumbled
- 1 medium pear
- 40 hazelnuts
- 4 tablespoons maple-Dijon vinaigrette

Directions:
1. Toast hazelnuts in a dry skillet for about 15 minutes, or toast on a baking sheet in a 350°F oven, stirring 2–3 times for both methods. Allow to cool and gently rub off the outer skin. Coarsely chop and set aside.
2. Toss dressing with the arugula and gorgonzola cheese and transfer to serving plates.
3. Arrange the pear slices in a fan on top and sprinkle with chopped hazelnuts.

Nutrition:
- **Calories:** 252
- **Fat:** 21 g
- **Net Carbs:** 8 g
- **Protein:** 8 g

3. Asian Roll-ups with Chicken and Peanut Sauce

Preparation Time: 30 minutes
Cooking Time: 20 minutes
Servings: 2
Ingredients:

- 2 chicken breast tenderloins - 1 ½ tablespoons tamari
- 1 tablespoon rice vinegar - 1 teaspoon minced ginger, divided
- 3 tbsp. liquid stevia - ½ avocado - ¼ cucumber with peel
- 2 ½ oz. cup jicama - 8 sprigs cilantro
- 2 sheets sushi nori - ½ tablespoon canola oil
- 1 ½ tablespoon natural creamy peanut butter
- 4 tablespoons water - ¾ teaspoon Sriracha sauce

Directions:

1. Place tamari, rice vinegar, ginger, and stevia in a plastic zip bag and shake to blend well. Add the chicken tenderloins to the marinade and set them aside.
2. While the chicken is marinating, prepare the vegetables. Slice the avocado into 8 long wedges. Cut the cucumber and jicama into sticks measuring about 3x1/8 inches. Divide ingredients into 4 equal portions. Set all aside on a cutting board, along with the sprigs of cilantro. Gently fold the nori sheets in half and then tear them in two; set all 4 sheets aside. Place the vegetable oil in a non-stick skillet over medium-high heat. Add the chicken, discarding the remaining marinade. Cook chicken until no longer pink in the center; about 3 minutes per side.
3. Place on the cutting board with the other ingredients and slice each tenderloin into 3 pieces (if you only had 3 tenderloins, cut into an amount that is easily divided by 4). Place a small dish of water next to the assembly line. Set aside.
4. In a small bowl combine the peanut butter, water, 1 ½ teaspoon tamari, remaining ½ teaspoon minced ginger, 3–4 drops stevia, and ¾ teaspoon Sriracha. Blend until all ingredients are incorporated, adjust seasonings to taste by adding more tamari, ginger, stevia, or sriracha.
5. **Assembly**: Place 1/2 sheet of nori on a flat surface. Place the sliced avocado, cucumber, jicama, and cilantro at a slight angle so they align with the corner of one end of the nori sheet with about 1/2-inch of the corner of the nori sheet sticking out. Dredge the chicken in the peanut sauce and place it on top of the vegetables. Roll, starting at the side where you placed the ingredients, then change direction slightly so that it creates a cone shape, with one end tightly rolled and the other end open. Dip your fingertips in the water bowl, and spread water on the nori sheet at the end corner of the wrap, hold it down a few seconds to seal the wrap in place. Repeat for remaining wraps. Use any remaining sauce for dipping.

Nutrition:

- **Calories:** 404 **Fat:** 23 g **Net Carbs:** 8 g **Protein:** 31 g

4. Baked Egg and Asparagus

Preparation Time: 5 minutes
Cooking Time: 10 minutes
Servings: 1
Ingredients:
- 4 small spears asparagus, woodsy end chopped off
- 2 eggs
- 1 tablespoon parmesan cheese
- ⅛ teaspoon garlic powder
- Pinch of fresh ground black pepper

Directions:
1. Preheat oven to 400°F
2. Grease a small oven-safe baking dish.
3. Steam the asparagus for 2 minutes.
4. Drain, rinse under cold water, and pat dry.
5. Arrange the asparagus in a circle around the baking dish. Crack in 2 eggs. Season with garlic powder, pepper.
6. Bake for 5 minutes. Remove from the oven. Sprinkle parmesan cheese over the top. Return to the oven for 3 minutes.
7. Serve immediately.

Nutrition:
- **Calories:** 471
- **Fat:** 40 g
- **Carbs:** 6 g
- **Protein:** 20.8 g
- **Dietary Fiber:** 4 g

5. Breakfast Tacos

Preparation Time: 10 minutes
Cooking Time: 15–20 minutes
Servings: 3
Ingredients:
- 1 cup shredded mozzarella cheese
- 6 eggs
- 2 tablespoons butter
- 3 bacon strips
- ½ avocado, thinly sliced
- ½ cup shredded cheddar cheese
- Pinch of salt and pepper

Directions:
1. Preheat oven to 375°F
2. Cook the bacon. Set aside.
3. You are going to make your very own cheese taco shells. Suspend a yardstick/ruler/long spoon between two items that prop it 6 inches from a counter.
4. Heat a skillet. Scoop half a cup of mozzarella cheese on the surface. Spread into a circle. Cook for 3 minutes until golden brown. Flip and cook on the other side. Lift the circle of cheese off the surface, drape it over a yardstick/ruler. Let it cool as you cook the others and the rest of the ingredients.
5. In a separate bowl, whisk the eggs. Season with salt and pepper. Melt butter in a skillet. Scramble the eggs.
6. **Prepare the tacos:** Place a slice of bacon in a cheese taco shell. Add a couple of spoons of cooked egg. Top with shredded cheddar cheese and sliced avocado.

Nutrition:
- **Calories:** 443
- **Fat:** 32 g
- **Carbs:** 7 g
- **Protein:** 3 g
- **Fiber:** 7 g
- **Dietary Fiber:** 27 g

6. Breakfast Burger

Preparation Time: 5 minutes
Cooking Time: 10–15 minutes
Servings: 6
Ingredients:
- 2 cups lean ground sausage
- 1 cup shredded pepper jack cheese
- 6 bacon slices
- 6 eggs
- 1 tablespoon PBfit® powder
- Pinch of salt and pepper

Directions:
1. Cook the bacon and set it aside.
2. In a bowl, combine the ground sausage, salt, and pepper. Form palm-sized patties.
3. In a separate bowl, combine PB Fit powder and 1 teaspoon of water. Stir until combined. Add a little more water for a runnier consistency. Set aside.
4. Cook the sausage patties. Once cooked on both sides, cover one side with pepper jack cheese. Let it melt.
5. Cook the eggs, sunny side up, or broken yolk, your preference.
6. Assemble the burgers: A sausage patty, slice of bacon, fried egg, dollop of PBfit® powder. Serve immediately.

Nutrition:
- **Calories:** 655
- **Fat:** 56 g
- **Carbs:** 5 g
- **Protein:** 30.5 g
- **Fiber:** 0.5 g
- **Net Carbs:** 3 g

7. Salmon and Egg Stuffed Avocados

Preparation Time: 15 minutes
Cooking Time: 20 minutes
Servings: 4
Ingredients:
- 4 avocados
- 4 oz. smoked salmon
- 8 eggs, organic
- Salt and black pepper
- Pinch of chili flakes
- Fresh dill to taste

Directions:
1. Preheat the oven to 425°F.
2. Cut the avocados in half and remove the seed.
3. If the hole from the pit is too small to hold an egg, scoop out enough to create the correct size.
4. Place the avocado halves on a cookie sheet; use strips of smoked salmon to line the hole left from the pit.
5. Using an egg separator, place a yolk on top of the salmon strips.
6. Spoon in as much egg white to each half as the hole will allow.
7. Add salt and pepper as desired.
8. Bake the avocados for 15–20 minutes; until the eggs are completely set.
9. Remove from the oven; sprinkle with chili flakes and fresh dill.
10. Serve the avocados warm.

Nutrition:
- **Calories:** 569
- **Total Carbs:** 18 g
- **Net Carbs:** 5 g
- **Fat:** 50 g
- **Protein:** 20 g

8. Cream Cheese Pancakes

Preparation Time: 10 minutes
Cooking Time: 10–15 minutes
Servings: 4
Ingredients:
- 4 oz. cream cheese
- 4 eggs, organic
- 4 teaspoons stevia
- 1 teaspoon cinnamon

Directions:
1. Coat a medium griddle or frying pan with cooking spray; heat the pan to medium.
2. Combine all the ingredients in a blender; blend at a high speed until the ingredients in a smooth mixture.
3. Let the ingredients sit for 2 minutes; the bubbles in the mixture will settle.
4. Pour ¼ of the mixture into the hot pan.
5. Cook the pancake for 2 minutes on one side (it will be golden).
6. Flip the pancake and cook it for 1 minute on the other side.
7. Remove the pancake from the pan with a spatula; place it on a plate and cover it to keep it warm.
8. Repeat steps with the remaining batter.
9. Serve the pancakes warm with any topping you choose

Nutrition:
- **Calories:** 163
- **Total Carbs:** 6 g
- **Net Carbs:** 3 g
- **Fat:** 14 g
- **Protein:** 7 g

9. Bacon, Egg & Cheese Casserole

Preparation Time: 15 minutes
Cooking Time: 15 minutes
Servings: 2
Ingredients:
- 12 eggs
- 6 bacon slices
- 4 oz. sour cream
- 4 oz. heavy cream
- 10 oz. cheddar cheese, shredded
- 1/3 cup chopped green onions
- Salt
- Pepper
- Cooking spray

Directions:
1. Preheat your oven to 350°F.
2. Fry the bacon in a skillet. Set aside on paper towels and cool. Crumble into bacon bits after cooling.
3. In a bowl, place the eggs, sour cream, heavy cream, salt, and pepper. Blend well with a hand mixer.
4. Prepare a baking dish or pan and spray with cooking spray.
5. Place a single layer of cheese in the pan. Cover the cheese with the egg mixture.
6. Now top everything with the crumbled bacon.
7. Bake in the oven for few minutes. Remove from the oven when the edges are browned and serve garnished with chopped green onions.

Nutrition:
- **Calories:** 437
- **Fat:** 38 g
- **Protein:** 43 g
- **Carbs:** 2 g

10. Vanilla and Marshmallow Smoothie

Preparation Time: 10 minutes
Cooking Time: 25 minutes
Servings: 2
Ingredients:
- ½ cup coconut milk
- 1 cup water
- 3 cups ice
- 2 tablespoons chia
- 1 teaspoon vanilla extract
- 2 tablespoons collage hydrosol
- Honey to taste

Directions:
1. Place the ingredients in your blender or food processor.
2. Blend until creamy smooth. Enjoy.

Nutrition:
- **Calories:** 257
- **Fat:** 18.7 g
- **Protein:** 8.1 g
- **Carbs:** 17.9 g

11. Broccoli Egg Muffins

Preparation Time: 10 minutes
Cooking Time: 5 minutes
Servings: 5
Ingredients:
- 1/3 cup green olives, chopped
- 5 large organic eggs
- 3 green onions, chopped
- 1 cup Parmesan cheese
- 3 tablespoons coconut milk, unsweetened
- ½ cup broccoli florets, chopped
- Salt and black pepper, to taste
- Cooking spray, for greasing
- 1 cup water

Directions:
1. Coat 3 custard cups with cooking spray.
2. In a mixing bowl, whisk the eggs together with the salt and pepper.
3. Stir in the onions, olives, coconut milk, cheese, and broccoli; mix well.
4. Pour 1/3 of the batter into each of the custard cups.
5. Place 1 cup of water in an Instant Pot; insert a trivet.
6. Put the custard cups on the trivet.
7. Close the lid of the Instant Pot and lock it.
8. Cook for 5 minutes under high pressure.
9. Turn the Instant Pot off when the timer beeps; use the quick release for the steam.
10. Once the steam has been released, open the lid of the Instant Pot.
11. Carefully remove the custard cups.
12. Serve the muffins hot.

Nutrition:
- **Calories:** 207
- **Total Carbs:** 9 g
- **Net Carbs:** 3 g
- **Fat:** 14 g
- **Protein:** 17 g

12. Raspberry Bread
Preparation Time: 30 minutes
Cooking Time: 25 minutes
Servings: 4
Ingredients:
- 2 cups almond flour
- 1/2 cup melted butter
- 1/2 cup almond milk
- 1 teaspoon vanilla extract
- 4 tablespoons stevia
- 1/3 cup raspberries
- 2 teaspoons dry yeast, dissolved in warm water
- Salt, pinch
- Cooking spray, for greasing
- 2 cups water

Directions:
1. Pour 1 cup of warm (not hot) water into a small bowl.
2. Sprinkle approximately 2 teaspoons of yeast over the water; let it sit for at least 15 minutes to fully dissolve the yeast.
3. In a medium bowl, combine the butter, vanilla extract, stevia, and yeast; stir until the ingredients are well-mixed.
4. Stir in the almond flour, almond milk, raspberries, and salt to create the batter.
5. Pour 1 cup of water into an Instant Pot; insert a trivet.
6. Put a piece of aluminum foil on the trivet that is large enough to go under the loaf pan and up both sides.
7. Coat the bottom and sides of a loaf pan with cooking spray.
8. Pour the batter into the loaf pan and place the loaf pan on the trivet.
9. Close the lid of the Instant Pot and lock it.
10. Cook for 25 minutes under high pressure.
11. Turn the Instant Pot off when the timer beeps; use the quick release for the steam.
12. Once the steam has been released, open the lid of the Instant Pot.
13. Remove the loaf pan from the Instant Pot using the aluminum foil on either side of the loaf pan to lift it out.
14. Let the bread sit for five minutes, then turn it out of the loaf pan onto a wire rack.
15. Allow the bread to cool thoroughly on the rack before slicing it.
16. Serve the bread alone or with a spread.

Nutrition:
- **Calories:** 369 **Total Carbs:** 4
- **Net Carbs:** 4 g **Fat:** 30 g **Protein:** 4 g

13. Ham and Cheddar Omelet

Preparation Time: 5 minutes
Cooking Time: 20 minutes
Servings: 5
Ingredients:
- 2 ham steaks
- 1 tablespoon butter
- ½ onion, diced
- 1 garlic clove, minced
- 7 eggs
- 1 cup shredded cheddar cheese
- ½ cup heavy cream
- Pinch of salt and pepper
- 1 tablespoon fresh chives, chopped

Directions:
1. Preheat oven to 400°F
2. Cook the ham steak, diced into cubes.
3. In a large bowl, combine the eggs, heavy cream, salt, and pepper. Whisk until combined. Add the cubed ham.
4. Using a skillet for the oven, melt the butter. Sauté onion and garlic for 2 minutes. Pour into the egg/ham mixture.
5. Bake 20 minutes, until golden brown.
6. Garnish with chopped chives.

Nutrition:
- **Calories:** 408
- **Fat:** 36 g
- **Carbs:** 7 g
- **Protein:** 16 g
- **Fiber:** 0.2 g
- **Net Carbs:** 5 g

14. Mini Pancake Donuts

Preparation Time: 5 minutes
Cooking Time: 3–5 minutes
Servings: 22
Ingredients:
- 6 tablespoons cream cheese
- 3 eggs
- 4 tablespoons almond flour
- 1 tablespoon coconut flour
- 1 teaspoon baking powder
- 1 teaspoon pure vanilla extract
- 4 tablespoons Erythritol
- 10 drops liquid stevia

Directions:
1. Using a hand blender, mix the cream cheese until smooth. Add one egg at a time, Blend after each egg until fully combined.
2. In a separate bowl, combine the almond flour, coconut flour, baking powder, Erythritol. Mix well. Add the dry ingredients slowly to the cream cheese. Blend until combined. Add the vanilla, liquid stevia. Stir until a batter forms.
3. Donut maker instructions: heat canola oil. Drop in the batter by full tablespoons. Cook 2 minutes, open lid, flip to the other side. Cook until golden brown.
4. Donut pan instructions: grease the pan. Bake in the oven at 350°F for 17–20 minutes, until golden brown.
5. Cool 5 minutes.

Nutrition:
- **Calories:** 31
- **Fat:** 7 g
- **Carbs:** 0.7 g
- **Protein:** 4 g
- **Fiber:** 0.3 g
- **Net Carbs:** 0.4 g

15. Pizza Waffles

Preparation Time: 10 minutes
Cooking Time: 3–5 minutes
Servings: 2
Ingredients:
- 4 eggs
- 1 tablespoon parmesan cheese
- 3 tablespoons almond flour
- 1 tablespoon psyllium husk powder
- 1 tablespoon bacon grease or canola oil
- 1 tablespoon baking powder
- 1 teaspoon Italian seasoning
- 14 slices pepperoni, diced
- Pinch of salt and pepper
- ½ cup tomato sauce
- ½ cup shredded cheddar cheese

Directions:
1. In a bowl, combine the eggs, parmesan cheese, almond flour, psyllium husk powder, baking powder, bacon grease or oil, Italian seasoning, pepperoni, salt, and pepper. Stir until a batter forms.
2. Heat waffle maker. Lightly brush with canola oil. Pour in ¼ to ½ cup of batter. Close waffle maker. Cook 10 minutes, or until golden brown.
3. Preheat oven to broil.
4. Remove waffles. Place on a baking sheet.
5. Spoon 1 tablespoon of tomato sauce over the waffle. Sprinkle cheddar cheese on top.
6. Place waffles under the broiler for 1–2 minutes until cheese melts.

Nutrition:
- **Calories:** 525
- **Fat:** 45 g
- **Carbs:** 5 g
- **Protein:** 29 g
- **Fiber:** 5 g
- **Net Carbs:** 0 g

16. Pancakes, Berries, Whipped Cream Breakfast

Preparation Time: 10 minutes
Cooking Time: 10 minutes
Servings: 1
Ingredients:
- 40 g blueberries
- 2 tablespoons cream cheese
- 2 eggs
- 20 ml double cream
- Pinch of ground cinnamon
- ¼ teaspoon Splenda® (or a sweetener of personal preference)
- 1 tsp. butter

Directions:
1. Beat the eggs into a blender then add the cinnamon, cream cheese, and sweetener.
2. Blend until thick, uniform liquid forms. Allow it to rest for 2 minutes for the bubbles to settle.
3. Pour ½ of the batter into the hot non-stick frying pan oiled with butter.
4. Allow the batter to cook until it turns to golden before flipping it over. This will take 3–4 minutes.
5. Repeat with the other half of the butter.
6. Whisk the double cream and once thickened well enough, top the pancakes with blueberries.

Nutrition:
- **Calories:** 382
- **Fat:** 28 g
- **Net Carbs:** 3 g
- **Protein:** 22 g

17. Eggs and Healthy Vegetables Fried in Coconut Oil

Preparation Time: 10 minutes
Cooking Time: 10 minutes
Servings: 1
Ingredients:
- ½ cup spinach
- Spices (salt and pepper), to taste
- ½ cup green beans
- 1/2 tbsp. coconut oil
- ½ cup carrots
- ½ cup broccoli
- ½ cup cauliflower
- 3–4 eggs

Directions:
1. Put the clean frypan over the fire, add some coconut oil to it, giving it some time to heat up.
2. Wash and chop the veggies up before dipping them in the hot coconut oil to fry.
3. If the veggies are frozen, let them thaw in the heat for a few minutes before cutting and eventually frying them up.
4. After a few minutes, beat the eggs up, emptying the contents into the frypan.
5. Add the spices.
6. Add the spinach (though it's optional in this case).
7. Continue to stir-fry the contents in the frypan until it's ready.

Nutrition:
- **Calories:** 80
- **Fat:** 5 g
- **Net Carbs:** 4 g
- **Protein:** 4 g

18. Protein Pancakes

Preparation Time: 5 minutes
Cooking Time: 10 minutes
Servings: 4
Ingredients:
- 1 tablespoon vanilla whey protein powder
- ¼ cup almond flour
- 3 tablespoons whole-grain soy flour
- 1 teaspoon baking powder
- 3 large-sized whole eggs
- ⅓ cup cottage cheese, creamed
- Butter for greasing

Directions:
1. In a bowl, combine almond meal,
2. Protein powder, baking powder, and soy flour. Stir.
3. In a separate bowl, whisk the eggs. Add the creamed cottage cheese. Stir until combined. Add to dry ingredients. Stir until combined.
4. On a large griddle/skillet, melt butter over the surface. Scoop out ¼ cup of batter. Cook 2–3 minutes per side, until golden brown.

Nutrition:
- **Calories:** 191
- **Fat:** 9 g
- **Carbs:** 4 g
- **Protein:** 20 g
- **Dietary Fiber:** 6 g

19. Almond and Coconut Mug Muffin

Preparation Time: 3 minutes
Cooking Time: 1 minute
Servings: 1
Ingredients:
- 2 tablespoons almond flour
- ⅓ tablespoon Sucralose-based sweetener
- ⅓ tablespoon organic high-fiber coconut flour
- ¼ teaspoon minced almonds
- Pinch of dried coconut
- ½ teaspoon cinnamon
- ¼ teaspoon baking powder
- ⅛ teaspoon salt
- 1 large egg
- 1 teaspoon extra virgin olive oil
- 1 tsp. Butter

Directions:
1. In a larger coffee mug, add the almond flour, sweetener, coconut flour, minced almond, and dried coconut, cinnamon, and baking powder, salt. Stir with a fork.
2. Crack in the egg. Pour into olive oil. Stir until combined.
3. Pop into the microwave. Cook for 1 minute. Cook at 15-second intervals if more time is required.
4. Top with butter and more minced almond. Use a spoon to dig out the goodness.

Nutrition:
- **Calories:** 207
- **Fat:** 18 g
- **Carbs:** 5 g
- **Protein:** 7 g
- **Dietary Fiber:** 3 g

CHAPTER 2:

Snacks, Sides, and Appetizers

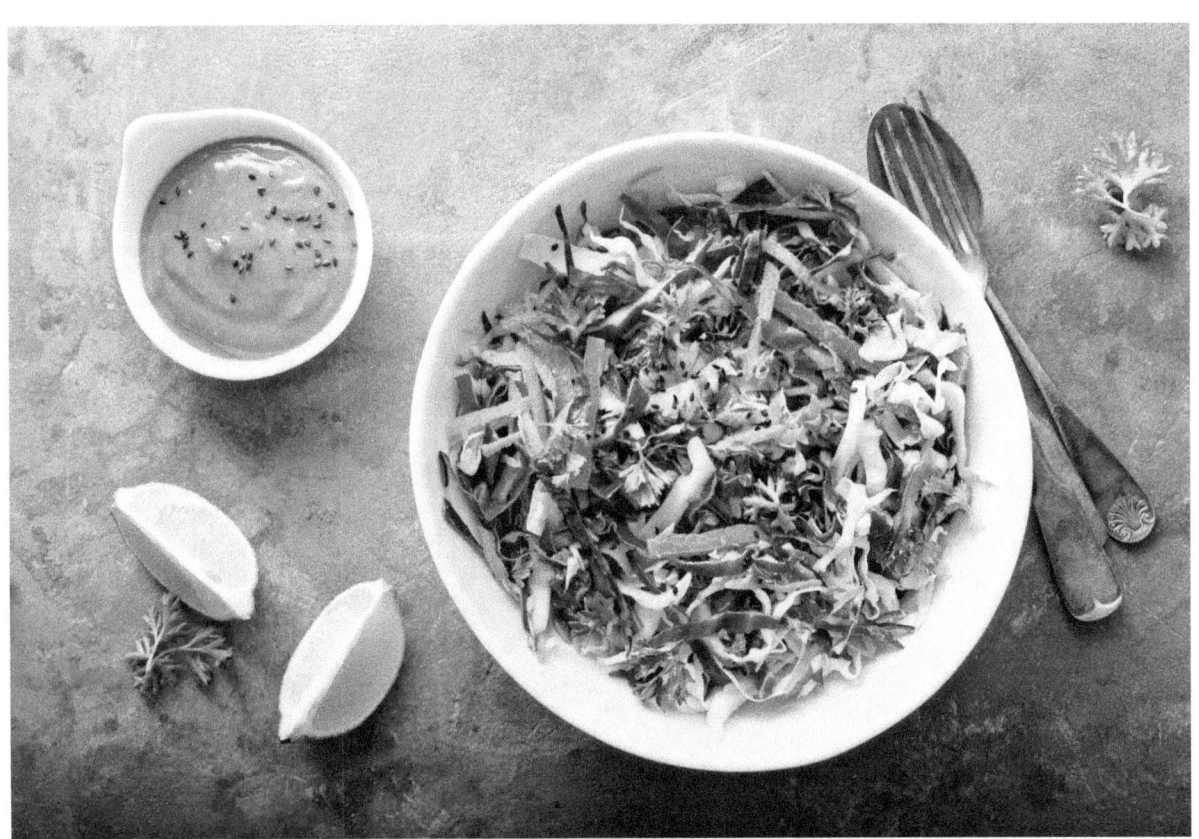

1. Caesar Salad Dressing

Preparation Time: 20 minutes
Cooking Time: 0 minutes
Servings: 2
Ingredients:
- 1 cup mayonnaise
- ¼ cup parmesan cheese, grated
- 2 tablespoons olive oil
- ¼ cup egg substitute
- 2 tablespoons water
- 1 tablespoon anchovy paste
- 1 tablespoon lemon juice
- 2 garlic cloves, crushed
- ¼ teaspoon dried parsley, chopped fine
- ½ teaspoon pepper, coarsely ground
- ¼ teaspoon salt
- 2 teaspoons sugar

Directions:
1. Start by combining all the ingredients required for the dish in a medium glass bowl.
2. With the help of an electric mixer, beat the ingredients above for just about 1 minute.
3. With the covered lid, refrigerate this for several hours.
4. That will increase the flavors of the dish.

Nutrition:
- **Carbs:** 17 g

2. Peanut Coleslaw

Preparation Time: 10 minutes
Cooking Time: 0 minutes
Servings: 2
Ingredients:
- 1 medium cabbage head
- 1 cup sour cream
- ½ cup peanuts
- 1/2 cup mayonnaise
- Sweetener (to taste)

Directions:
1. Start with chopping the cabbage semi-fine. Now process peanuts.
2. Add sour cream, mayo, and sweetener into the mix.
3. Combine with cabbage and peanuts.
4. Keep it for several hours in the fridge to blend flavors. You can also garnish it with a few whole peanuts.

Nutrition:
- **Carbs:** 26 g

3. Pecan and Gorgonzola Salad

Preparation Time: 10 minutes
Cooking Time: 0 minutes
Servings: 2
Ingredients:
- 6 cups lettuce leaf
- ½ cup Gorgonzola cheese
- ½ cup pecan pieces
- 3 tbsp. olive oil/balsamic vinegar
- Salt to taste
- Pepper to taste
- 1 tsp. butter

Directions:
1. Start with toasting the pecan pieces with some amount of butter.
2. Make sure that the toast will not get burned as it is very soft.
3. Now combine all the other ingredients with the toasted pecan pieces and toss well.
4. Add the seasoning of olive oil, salt, and pepper, and toss it again. The dish is ready for serving.

Nutrition:
- **Calories:** 110
- **Saturated fat:** 0.8 g
- **Total Carbs:** 16 g
- **Sugar:** 3 g
- **Protein:** 6 g

4. Pepper Ranch Salad Dressing

Preparation Time: 10 minutes
Cooking Time: 0 minutes
Servings: 2
Ingredients:
- 2 tablespoons sour cream
- 2 teaspoons heavy cream
- 1 tablespoon parmesan cheese, grated
- Pepper to taste, freshly ground
- 1 teaspoon ranch dressing

Directions:
1. Combine all the required ingredients all together in a big bowl and chill for several hours to set before serving.

Nutrition:
- **Carbs:** 2 g

5. Oven-Baked Carrot Fries

Preparation Time: 15 minutes
Cooking Time: 20 minutes
Servings: 2
Ingredients:
- 1 1/2 lbs. carrots
- 1 teaspoon sugar
- 2 tablespoons olive oil
- 1/2 teaspoon salt
- 2 tablespoons fresh rosemary, finely chopped
- 1 pinch pepper

Directions:
1. Heat oven to 425°F. Line a shallow pan with foil.
2. Using a sharp knife, slice away the tip and end of each carrot; peel each completely.
3. Cut carrots in half crosswise, then cut lengthwise, then cut lengthwise again.
4. In a mixing bowl, combine the carrot sticks, olive oil, rosemary, sugar, salt, and pepper. Stir until all are evenly coated.
5. Place carrots in the pan, spreading sticks out as much as possible. Bake for 20 minutes or until carrots are tender.
6. Serve hot or at room temperature.

Nutrition:
- **Calories:** 136.3
- **Sugars:** 8.9 g
- **Dietary Fiber:** 4.9 g
- **Protein:** 1.6 g

6. Zesty Baked Fries

Preparation Time: 10 minutes
Cooking Time: 50 minutes
Servings: 2
Ingredients:
- ¼ cup grated parmesan cheese
- 1 tablespoon olive oil
- 2 teaspoons basil
- 1 teaspoon oregano
- 1 teaspoon garlic powder
- 4 medium red potatoes
- Cooking spray

Directions:
1. Mix the first five ingredients.
2. Cut potatoes in the sticks.
3. Toss potatoes with cheese mixture.
4. Place on a baking sheet coated with cooking spray.
5. Spray potatoes lightly with cooking spray.
6. Bake at 425°F for 15 minutes, turn potatoes over, and bake 15 more minutes, until crispy.

Nutrition:
- **Calories:** 312
- **Total Fat:** 15 g
- **Saturated fat:** 2.3 g
- **Protein:** 3.4 g

7. Cauliflower Mushroom Risotto

Preparation Time: 10 minutes
Cooking Time: 10 minutes
Servings: 2
Ingredients:
- 1 tablespoon olive oil
- 2 garlic cloves, minced
- 4 baby Bella mushrooms, diced
- 1 cup chicken broth
- 2 cups riced cauliflower
- ¼ cup parmesan cheese
- ¼ cup heavy cream
- 1 teaspoon tarragon
- Pinch of salt and pepper

Directions:
1. In a blender, process the cauliflower until rice-like consistency.
2. In a skillet, heat the olive oil. Sauté the garlic and mushrooms for 3 minutes.
3. Pour in the chicken broth and cauliflower. Stir well. Simmer 5 minutes.
4. Once the liquid has cooked away, add the parmesan cheese and tarragon, salt, and pepper. Stir well. Stir in the cream. Keep stirring until the cheese has melted.
5. Serve hot.

Nutrition:
- **Calories:** 245.5
- **Fat:** 20 g
- **Carbs:** 8.5 g
- **Protein:** 7 g
- **Fiber:** 2.5 g
- **Net Carbs:** 6 g

8. Coconut Orange Creamsicle Fat Bombs

Preparation Time: 2–3 minutes
Cooking Time: 10 minutes
Servings: 2
Ingredients:
- ½ cup coconut oil
- ½ cup heavy whipping cream
- ¼ cup cream cheese
- 1 teaspoon orange-vanilla Mio®
- 10 drops liquid Stevia

Directions:
1. Add the coconut oil to a blender. Pulse until smooth.
2. Add the whipped cream. Pulse until combined.
3. Add the cream cheese. Pulse until smooth.
4. Add the orange Mio® and Stevia. Pulse until smooth.
5. Spoon the mixture into a silicone tray mold or ice cube tray. Freeze 3 hours.
6. Pop-out to eat. Store uneaten bombs in a bag in the freezer.

Nutrition:
- **Calories:** 176
- **Fat:** 20 g
- **Carbs:** 0.7 g
- **Protein:** 0.8 g
- **Fiber:** 0 g
- **Net Carbs:** 0.7 g

9. Corndog Muffins

Preparation Time: 10 minutes
Cooking Time: 15 minutes
Servings: 4
Ingredients:
- ½ cup blanched almond flour
- ½ cup flaxseed meal
- 1 tablespoon psyllium husk powder
- 3 tablespoons swerve® sweetener
- ¼ teaspoon salt
- ¼ teaspoon baking powder
- ¼ cup melted butter
- 1 egg
- ¼ cup coconut milk
- ⅓ cup sour cream
- 3 all-beef hot dogs

Directions:
1. Preheat oven to 375°F
2. In a bowl, add the almond flour, flaxseed, psyllium husk powder, granulated sweetener, salt, and baking powder. Whisk together.
3. In a separate bowl, combine the egg and coconut milk. Whisk together. Add the butter. Stir until combined. Add the sour cream. Stir until combined.
4. Add the dry ingredients to the wet ingredients. Stir until a smooth batter forms.
5. Grease a 12 mini muffin tin.
6. Slice the hot dogs into four.
7. Fill the muffin cup halfway. Add the sliced hot dog to the batter.
8. Bake 12 minutes.
9. Then broil for 1–2 minutes until golden brown. Serve.

Nutrition:
- **Calories:** 78.5
- **Fat:** 6.8 g
- **Carbs:** 2.1 g
- **Protein:** 2.4 g
- **Fiber:** 1.5 g
- **Net Carbs:** 0.7 g

10. Layered Fried Queso Blanco

Preparation Time: 10 minutes
Cooking Time: 10 minutes
Servings: 2
Ingredients:
- ½ cup Queso Blanco
- 1½ tablespoons olive oil
- Pinch red pepper flakes or salt and pepper

Directions:
1. Cut the cheese into cubes. Chill in the freezer as you heat the oil.
2. In a skillet, heat the olive oil. Once the pan is hot, add the cubes of cheese.
3. As it cooks, it will melt. Once it is golden brown on one side, flip it over. Press down against the cheese to flatten it slightly and push out the oil. Once it is golden brown on both sides, tilt the edges against the pan and cook until golden brown. It will seal the cheese into a square.
4. Remove from pan. Place on paper towel. Pat lightly. Slice into cubes again.
5. Sprinkle red pepper flakes or salt and pepper over the cubes. Serve immediately.

Nutrition:
- **Calories:** 525
- **Fat:** 43 g
- **Carbs:** 4 g
- **Protein:** 30 g
- **Fiber:** 2 g
- **Net Carbs:** 2 g

11. Pineapple Slaw

Preparation Time: 10 minutes
Cooking Time: 0 minutes
Servings: 2
Ingredients:
- 2 cups cabbage, shredded finely
- ¼ cup green peppers, diced finely
- ½ cup pineapple in juice, crushed drained
- 2 tablespoons onion
- 2 tablespoons mayonnaise
- 1 teaspoon finely chopped Stevia
- ¼ teaspoon celery seed salt to taste
- Sugar to taste
- Pepper to taste

Directions:
1. Combine pineapple with all types of veggies ingredients required for the dish. Toss well and mix the remaining ingredients all together.
2. Again toss and mix them well. Chill for several hours and mix also and serve cold.

Nutrition:
- **Calories:** 638
- **Protein:** 47.6 g
- **Fat:** 29.21 g
- **Carbs:** 50.28 g

12. Yummilicious Ginger Flan

Preparation Time: 15 minutes
Cooking Time: 40 minutes
Servings: 6
Ingredients:
- 3 egg yolks (from large eggs)
- 2 large whole eggs
- 1 cup tap water
- 3 teaspoon ginger
- 1 ½ cups heavy whipped cream
- 6 packets sucralose-based sugar sweetener
- 1 teaspoon vanilla extract

Directions:
1. Pre-heat oven to 350°F. Fill a roasting pan halfway with boiling water and place it on the center shelf in the oven.
2. In a blender, add the whole eggs, egg yolks, tap water, whipped cream, vanilla extract, ginger, and sugar substitute. Combine until a smooth mixture is formed.
3. Use a sieve to pour the mixture into a 1-quart baking dish. Gently, place the dish in a roasting pan. Bake for about half an hour or until a knife put in the center comes out clean.
4. Remove and let it cool on a wire rack. Spray a plastic wrap sheet with a cooking spray, lay it directly over the baking dish, and freeze it for about 3 hours in the refrigerator.
5. Take away the plastic wrap and remove flan from the mold by placing a plate over the top and flipping it onto a table to make sure the pan is now upside down on the plate. Serve.

Nutrition:
- **Carbs:** 5 g
- **Fat:** 25 g
- **Protein:** 7 g
- **Calories:** 264

13. Atkins Coffee Eggnog

Preparation Time: 5 minutes
Cooking Time: 0 minutes
Servings: 4
Ingredients:
- 1 teaspoon sucralose-based sugar substitute
- ½ teaspoon vanilla extract
- 1 cup decaffeinated coffee
- 1 cup whipped heavy cream
- 3 fl. oz. rum (optional)
- 2 large whole eggs
- 1/8 teaspoon ground cinnamon

Directions:
1. In a medium mixing bowl, beat the whole eggs and sugar substitute. Add vanilla extract, whipped cream, coffee, and rum; combine well to form a smooth mixture.
2. Top with cinnamon and enjoy your coffee eggnog.

Nutrition:
- **Carbs:** 1 g
- **Fat:** 25 g
- **Protein:** 4 g
- **Calories:** 308

14. Beet-Pickled Deviled Eggs

Preparation Time: 10 minutes (Not including brining time)
Cooking Time: 20 minutes
Servings: 12 pieces
Ingredients:
- 6 large eggs
- 1 cup apple cider vinegar
- 16 oz. jar pickled beets
- ⅓ cup brown sugar
- 1 tablespoon whole peppercorns
- 1 teaspoon salt
- 2 tablespoons olive oil
- 1 tablespoon Dijon mustard
- 1 tablespoon mayonnaise
- ½ teaspoon curry powder
- Freshly ground black pepper to desired taste
- Chopped fresh rosemary leaves to garnish
- ½ cup white vinegar

Directions:
1. Hard boil the eggs and then let them cool. Peel off the shells and set them aside.
2. Pour the jar of beets into a large bowl, then add apple cider vinegar, peppercorns, sugar, and salt. Stir to combine well. This is your brine.
3. Carefully place peeled eggs into the brine and refrigerate for at least 12 hours. No more than 3 days in the brine.
4. Remove from the brine solution and cut each egg in half, top to bottom. Scoop out the yolk of each egg carefully and place it in a bowl. Mash all the egg yolk.
5. Add the white vinegar, mayonnaise, olive oil, curry powder, and mustard to the egg yolk and mix everything well to combine. Everything should blend together smoothly. Add some pepper and salt for the desired flavoring and mix well again.
6. Take the egg yolk mixture and distribute evenly between all the formed egg whites using a spoon.
7. Garnish with the chopped rosemary and they are ready to serve. This is a great snack.

Nutrition:
- **Calories:** 178
- **Total Fats:** 5 g
- **Protein:** 3 g
- **Carbs:** 17 g

15. Cashew Bread

Preparation Time: 60 minutes
Cooking Time: 20 minutes
Servings: 16 slices

Ingredients:
- 5 large eggs
- 1 tablespoon apple cider vinegar
- 1 cup cashew butter
- ¾ teaspoon baking soda
- ¼ teaspoon sea salt

Directions:
1. Turn on the oven to 350°F and preheat.
2. Add eggs and cashew butter to a food processor. Pulse until smooth.
3. Add in the apple cider vinegar and process well.
4. Add in the sea salt and baking soda and process one more time.
5. Grease a 9x5 inch loaf dish. Pour in the contents of the food processor.
6. Place in the oven and cook for 45 minutes.
7. Take out of the oven and allow the bread to cool down on a rack for at least 1–2 hours.
8. Slice the bread and now it is ready to serve.

Nutrition:
- **Calories:** 178
- **Total Fats:** 5 g
- **Proteins:** 3 g
- **Carbs:** 17 g

CHAPTER 3:

Lunch

1. Fish Strips, Basil & Feta Salad

Preparation Time: 5 minutes
Cooking Time: 40 minutes
Servings: 4
Ingredients:
- 1 fish fillet, sliced into strips
- Salt and pepper to taste
- 1 egg, beaten
- 1 cup coconut shreds
- 1 tablespoon coconut oil
- ½ cup olive oil
- 1 garlic clove
- 4 oz. feta cheese
- 4 tablespoons sundried tomatoes, chopped
- 4 oz. black olives
- 6 cups mixed greens

Directions:
1. Season the fish strips with salt and pepper.
2. Dip into the egg and coat with shredded coconut.
3. Pour the coconut oil into the Instant Pot and set it to sauté.
4. Cook until golden on both sides.
5. Chop the breaded fish and set it aside.
6. Arrange the mixed greens in a salad bowl.
7. Top with tomatoes, olives, and feta.
8. Puree the garlic and olive oil to make the dressing.
9. Sprinkle chopped fish strip on top and drizzle dressing.

Nutrition:
- **Calories:** 254 **Total Fat:** 13 g
- **Sodium:** 244mg **Total Carbs:** 15 g
- **Dietary Fiber:** 5 g **Total Sugars:** 5 g **Protein:** 4 g

2. Salmon & Bok Choy

Preparation Time: 5 minutes
Cooking Time: 30 minutes
Servings: 4
Ingredients:
- 2 tablespoons organic tamari
- 1 tablespoon lemon juice
- 12 oz. salmon
- 2 tablespoons olive oil
- 1 ½ Chinese cabbage head, sliced in half
- 6 oz. mushrooms
- ½ tablespoons butter
- Salt and pepper to taste

Directions:
1. In a bowl, mix the tamari and lemon juice.
2. Pour half into another bowl and set aside.
3. Marinate the salmon for 30 minutes.
4. Place the salmon in the Instant Pot.
5. Seal the pot and choose the manual mode.
6. Cook at high pressure for 3 minutes.
7. Release the pressure quickly.
8. Switch the pot to sauté.
9. Pour in the olive oil.
10. Add the butter.
11. Cook the cabbage and mushrooms.
12. Season with salt and pepper.
13. Add the salmon and the remaining marinade.
14. Simmer for 5 minutes.

Nutrition:
- **Calories:** 242
- **Total Fat:** 15 g
- **Sodium:** 758 mg
- **Total Carbs:** 9 g
- **Dietary Fiber:** 7 g
- **Total Sugars:** 7 g
- **Protein:** 26 g

3. Fish Fillet with Capers & Tomatoes

Preparation Time: 3 minutes
Cooking Time: 20 minutes
Servings: 6

Ingredients:
- 1 tablespoon olive oil
- 1 onion, chopped
- 10 pieces black olives
- 1 teaspoon garlic
- 2 tablespoons capers, rinsed and drained
- 2 tomatoes, chopped
- 4 oz. red table wine
- 1/8 teaspoon crushed red pepper flakes
- 4 tablespoons butter

Directions:
1. Pour the oil into the Instant Pot.
2. Add the onion and olives.
3. Cook for 3 minutes.
4. Add the garlic, capers, and tomatoes.
5. Cook for 2 minutes.
6. Pour in the red wine and season with the red pepper flakes.
7. Close the pot.
8. Set it to manual.
9. Cook at high pressure for 2 minutes.
10. Release the pressure naturally.
11. Stir in the butter and simmer until the sauce has thickened.

Nutrition:
- **Calories:** 408
- **Total Fat:** 25 g
- **Sodium:** 930mg
- **Total Carbs:** 30.1 g
- **Dietary Fiber:** 9 g
- **Total Sugars:** 2 g
- **Protein:** 29 g

4. Shrimp Scampi

Preparation Time: 10 minutes
Cooking Time: 5 to 10 minutes
Servings: 4
Ingredients:
- 2 tablespoons extra virgin olive oil
- 2 tablespoons butter
- 1 tablespoon minced garlic
- 2 shallots, minced
- ½ cup dry white wine
- 1½ pounds extra-large shrimp, peeled
- Sea salt
- Freshly ground black pepper
- ½ lemon juice
- ¼ cup minced fresh flat-leaf parsley

Directions:
1. Heat a large skillet over medium heat until hot, then pour in the oil and melt the butter. Tilt to coat the bottom.
2. Add the garlic and shallots, and cook for about 3 minutes, or until they begin to soften.
3. Add the wine, and cook for about 2 minutes to cook off some of the alcohol.
4. Add the shrimp and sauté for 2 to 3 minutes, stirring and flipping to cook on all sides, or until just cooked through.
5. Season with salt and pepper, sprinkle with lemon juice, and garnish with parsley.

Nutrition:
- **Calories:** 312
- **Fat:** 15 g
- **Saturated Fat:** 5 g
- **Sodium:** 485 mg
- **Total Carbs:** 3 g
- **Net Carbs:** 3 g
- **Fiber:** 0 g
- **Sugar:** 0 g
- **Protein:** 36 g

5. Chicken with Peanut Sauce

Preparation Time: 5 minutes
Cooking Time: 45 minutes
Servings: 4
Ingredients:

- 8 oz. chicken tenderloin
- 1 ½ tablespoons tamari, divided
- 1 tablespoon rice vinegar
- 1 teaspoon ginger, divided
- 4 drops liquid Stevia
- 1 tablespoon olive oil
- 4 tablespoons water
- 2 cups creamy peanut butter
- 3/4 teaspoon hot sauce
- ½ avocado, sliced into strips
- ¼ cucumber, sliced into strips
- 8 sprigs cilantro

Directions:

1. Soak the chicken tenderloins in 1 tablespoon tamari, rice vinegar, half of the ginger, and liquid stevia for 30 minutes.
2. Choose the sauté setting in the Instant Pot.
3. Pour in the oil.
4. Brown the chicken on both sides.
5. In a bowl, combine the water, peanut butter, hot sauce, remaining tamari, and remaining ginger.
6. Pour the mixture into the pot and simmer for 5 minutes.
7. Serve with the avocado and cucumber slices, garnish with cilantro.

Nutrition:

- **Calories:** 436
- **Total Fat:** 37 g
- **Saturated Fat:** 6 g
- **Cholesterol:** 5 mg
- **Sodium:** 522 mg
- **Total Carbs:** 16 g
- **Dietary Fiber:** 8 g
- **Total Sugars:** 4 g
- **Protein:** 12 g
- **Potassium:** 516 mg

6. Chicken with Onion & Fennel

Preparation Time: 3 minutes
Cooking Time: 20 minutes
Servings: 4
Ingredients:
- 16 oz. chicken thigh
- Salt and pepper to taste
- 1 tablespoon olive oil
- 1 bulb fennel
- 1 onion, sliced into rings
- 2 cherry tomatoes, sliced in half
- 2 tablespoons butter
- 1 garlic clove, crushed
- 1 teaspoon thyme
- 1 teaspoon tarragon
- 1 tablespoon red wine vinegar
- 1/4 cup water

Directions:
1. Season the chicken with salt and pepper.
2. Add the oil to the Instant Pot.
3. Set it to sauté.
4. Brown the chicken on both sides.
5. Remove and set aside.
6. Add the onion and fennel into the pot.
7. Season with salt and pepper.
8. Cook until soft.
9. Add the rest of the ingredients.
10. Put the chicken back to the pot.
11. Cover the pot.
12. Set it to manual.
13. Cook at high pressure for 7 minutes.
14. Release the pressure naturally.
15. Serve warm.

Nutrition:
- **Calories:** 340 **Total Fat:** 18 g
- **Saturated Fat:** 5 g **Cholesterol:** 116 mg
- **Sodium:** 174 mg **Total Carbs:** 8 g
- **Dietary Fiber:** 3 g **Total Sugars:** 8 g
- **Protein:** 35 g **Potassium:** 718 mg

7. Rosemary Chicken

Preparation Time: 2 minutes
Cooking Time: 20 minutes
Servings: 2
Ingredients:
- 20 oz. chicken thigh
- 1 teaspoon rosemary
- Salt and pepper to taste
- 3 tablespoons olive oil
- 1 cup chicken broth
- 4 oz. white wine
- ½ cup onion, chopped
- 8 oz. mushroom

Directions:
1. Season the chicken with rosemary, salt, and pepper.
2. Add the olive oil to the Instant Pot.
3. Set it to sauté.
4. Add the onion and mushroom and cook for 1 minute.
5. Take out of the pot and set aside.
6. Add the chicken and cook until brown on both sides.
7. Pour in the chicken broth and white wine, and toss to coat evenly.
8. Close the pot and choose the manual mode.
9. Cook at high pressure for 5 minutes.
10. Release the pressure naturally.
11. Take the chicken out and set it aside.
12. Drizzle the cooking liquid and top the chicken with the onion and mushrooms before serving.

Nutrition:
- **Calories:** 411
- **Total Fat:** 26 g
- **Saturated Fat:** 5 g
- **Cholesterol:** 126 mg
- **Sodium:** 318 mg
- **Total Carbs:** 4 g
- **Dietary Fiber:** 1 g
- **Total Sugars:** 2 g
- **Protein:** 42 g
- **Potassium:** 629 mg

8. Moroccan Beef Lettuce Wraps

Preparation Time: 30 minutes
Cooking Time: 10 hours
Servings: 2
Ingredients:
- 12 oz. beef roast, trimmed and cut into bite-size pieces
- 1 cup sliced white onions
- 1 teaspoon sea salt
- 4 tablespoons garam masala,
- 10 large lettuce leaves for wrapping

Directions:
1. Grease a 4-quart slow-cooker and add all the ingredients apart from the lettuce.
2. Cover and seal slow-cooker with its lid.
3. Set the cooking timer for 8 hours and allow you to cook at a low heat setting.
4. Remove the beef and shred it using forks. Place the meat back in the slow cooker and continue cooking for another 2 hours.
5. Serve warm, wrapped in the lettuce leaves.

Nutrition:
- **Calories:** 209
- **Carbs:** 0.7 g
- **Net Carbs:** 0.7 g
- **Fat:** 9.5 g
- **Protein:** 30.4 g

9. Steak Fajitas

Preparation Time: 10 minutes
Cooking Time: 50 minutes
Servings: 2
Ingredients:
- 1 red and one green bell pepper, de-seeded and sliced
- 1 white onion, peeled and sliced
- 2 tablespoons fajita seasoning
- 20 oz. tomato salsa, sugar-free
- Cheese, shredded
- Sour cream

Directions:
1. Grease a 4-quart slow-cooker with a non-stick cooking spray and then pour the salsa in.
2. Place the peppers and onion on top, and sprinkle with the fajita seasoning.
3. Stir until mixed well, then cover and seal the slow-cooker with its lid.
4. Set the cooking timer for 3 to 4 hours and cook at a high heat setting.
5. Serve with shredded cheese and sour cream.

Nutrition:
- **Calories:** 222
- **Carbs:** 5 g
- **Net Carbs:** 4 g
- **Fat:** 12 g
- **Protein:** 23 g

10. Beef and Eggplant

Preparation Time: 30 minutes
Cooking Time: 4.5 hours
Servings: 2
Ingredients:
2/3 lb. ground beef
1 can chopped tomatoes
2/3 medium-sized eggplant, de-stemmed
1 tablespoon Lebanese Spice Blend
2/3 cup shredded mozzarella cheese
Cooking spray
Salt
Black pepper
Parsley, for garnish

Directions:
1. Cut the eggplant into large chunks and add to a 4-quart slow-cooker, greased with non-stick cooking spray.
2. Stir together the ground beef and the spice blend, and season with salt and ground black pepper. Place this over the eggplant.
3. Pour over the chopped tomato and then place the lid on the slow-cooker.
4. Set the cooking timer for 4 hours and allow you to cook at a low heat setting.
5. Add the shredded mozzarella and cook for a further 30 minutes until the cheese is melted.
6. Garnish with parsley to serve.

Nutrition:
- **Calories:** 209
- **Carbs:** 8.1 g
- **Net Carbs:** 7.4 g
- **Fat:** 12.8 g
- **Protein:** 15.9 g

11. Barbecue Pulled Beef

Preparation Time: 30 minutes
Cooking Time: 4 hours
Servings: 2
Ingredients:
- 12 oz. beef pot roast, trimmed and cut into bite-sized pieces
- 1 teaspoon minced garlic
- 1 teaspoon onion powder
- 1/4 cup apple cider vinegar
- 3/4 cup tomato ketchup, sugar-free
- Cooking spray
- A pinch of salt and black pepper
- 8 oz. portobello mushrooms

Directions:
1. Grease a 4-quart slow-cooker with a non-stick cooking spray.
2. Mix all the ingredients, apart from the beef, and place the mixture in the slow-cooker.
3. Add the beef pieces and season with a pinch of salt and ground black pepper.
4. Cover and seal the slow-cooker with its lid, setting the cooking timer for 4 hours, and allowing cooking at a high heat setting.
5. Shred the meat with forks and serve between roasted Portobello mushroom caps.

Nutrition:
- **Calories:** 380
- **Carbs:** 6 g
- **Net Carbs:** 5.2 g
- **Fat:** 15 g
- **Protein:** 49 g

12. Pumpkin Soup with Coconut and Curry

Preparation Time: 15 minutes
Cooking Time: 25 minutes
Servings: 2
Ingredients:

- 800 grams sliced pumpkin cubes
- 1–2 garlic cloves
- 2 teaspoon curry powder
- Salt and pepper
- 400 ml chicken broth
- 400 ml water
- 200 ml coconut milk
- Butter
- Onion

Directions:

1. Melt a piece of butter in a large soup pot.
2. Heat the chicken broth in another pan at the same time.
3. Cut the onion into small pieces and fry gently in the pan for 5 minutes.
4. Add the diced pumpkin and fry it until softer.
5. Add the garlic, curry powder, salt, and pepper to the onion and cook together for 1 minute.
6. Simultaneously, heat the coconut milk in a separate pan and stir in occasionally.
7. Add the chicken stock and water to the whole and mix well.
8. Put the heat on a low.
9. Boil slowly for 20 minutes and stir occasionally.
10. Put the soup in the blender together with the coconut milk and mix until smooth.
11. Then add it to the soup pan again and heat it until it is warm enough to be served.

Nutrition:

- **Calories:** 335
- **Carbs:** 27 g
- **Fat:** 18 g
- **Protein:** 23 g

13. Quick Seafood Chowder

Preparation Time: 20 minutes
Cooking Time: 15 minutes
Servings: 2
Ingredients:
- 1 teaspoon garlic
- 6 tablespoons shallots, chopped
- 4 tablespoons light olive oil
- 2 stalks celery, chopped
- 12 cherry tomatoes
- 6 tablespoons clam juice, all-natural
- 2 cups chicken broth, organic and homemade
- 1/6 teaspoon Italian seasoning
- 1/8 teaspoon black pepper
- 1 lb. shrimp
- 4 oz. blue crab
- 8 oz. clams

Directions:
1. Heat the oil in a large sauté pan or skillet.
2. Using medium heat, sauté the garlic and shallots for approximately 2 minutes (the shallots should be translucent and the garlic fragrant).
3. Add in the celery, tomatoes, clam juice, and broth, continually stirring; season with pepper and Italian seasoning.
4. Simmer for 3 minutes, stirring occasionally.
5. Stir in the shrimp, crab, and clams.
6. Bring the mixture to a simmer and cook for 5 minutes (the shrimp should be pink and firm); stir occasionally.
7. Remove to a serving bowl.
8. Serve warm.

Nutrition:
- **Calories:** 484
- **Total Carbs:** 28.2 g
- **Net Carbs:** 23.3 g
- **Fat:** 19 g
- **Protein:** 38 g

14. Atkins Diet Soup

Preparation Time: 25 minutes
Cooking Time: 35 minutes
Servings: 2
Ingredients:
- 3 bacon slices, chopped
- 2 teaspoons olive oil
- 1/3 cup onion, chopped
- 1 tablespoon fresh garlic, minced
- 1/2 cup sundried tomatoes, chopped
- 1/2 cup sliced white mushrooms
- 10 cups chicken stock
- 2 cups water
- 3 cups celery root, peeled and chopped
- 5 cups cooked chicken breast, chopped
- 1 cup yellow squash, sliced
- ½ cup green beans cut into 1 inch
- 5 cups Swiss chard, chopped
- 3 tablespoons red wine vinegar
- ¼ cup fresh basil, chopped
- Salt and freshly ground black pepper to taste

Directions:
1. Using a large soup pot, cook the bacon and olive oil for 2 minutes on medium heat.
2. Stir in the onions, sundried tomatoes, garlic, and mushrooms.
3. Cook for 6 minutes, stirring occasionally.
4. Add the water and stock, stir to mix.
5. Stir in the celery root and chicken.
6. Simmer for 15 minutes, stirring occasionally.
7. Add the squash, green beans, and Swiss chard.
8. Simmer for 10 minutes, stirring occasionally.
9. Stir in the red wine vinegar; add salt and pepper to taste.
10. Stir in the fresh basil before serving.
11. Serve.

Nutrition:
- **Calories:** 360
- **Total Carbs:** 22.2 g
- **Net Carbs:** 17.4 g
- **Fat:** 13 g
- **Protein:** 38 g

15. Blue Cheese and Bacon Soup

Preparation Time: 10 minutes
Cooking Time: 35 minutes
Servings: 2

Ingredients:
- 4 medium bacon slices
- 3 tablespoons butter
- 1 leek, chopped
- 2 cups mushroom pieces and stems
- 1 cup cauliflower
- 25 oz. can chicken broth
- 1/2 cup tap water
- 3 oz. blue cheese

Directions:
1. Cook the bacon over medium heat in a skillet or griddle.
2. Cook until the bacon is crispy on one side; flip the bacon over and cook until it is crisp all the way through.
3. Remove the bacon to a paper towel; pat it to remove any excess fat.
4. When the bacon is cold, crumble it and set it aside.
5. In the meantime, melt the butter in a large soup pot.
6. Add the leek, mushrooms, and cauliflower.
7. Stir the ingredients together.
8. Cover the pot and cook the vegetables for 5 minutes, stirring occasionally.
9. Pour in the chicken broth and water; bring the pot to a boil.
10. Reduce the heat; cover and simmer for 10 minutes (the vegetables should be very tender).
11. Remove the soup from the stove and puree it in a blender or food processor; when pureeing the last batch of soup, add the blue cheese.
12. Return the soup to the soup pot on the stove.
13. Heat until warmed through in low heat, if necessary.
14. Pour into bowls and top with crumbled bacon.
15. Serve.

Nutrition:
- **Calories:** 331
- **Total Carbs:** 10.4 g
- **Net Carbs:** 7.7 g
- **Fat:** 24 g
- **Protein:** 20 g

16. Versatile Vegetable Soup

Preparation Time: 15 minutes
Cooking Time: 25–30 minutes
Servings: 2
Ingredients:
- 4 tablespoons olive oil
- 1 stalk celery
- 1/2 teaspoon ground thyme, dried
- 1 teaspoon garlic, minced
- 2 small zucchini
- 1/4 cup green snap beans
- 1/4 teaspoon salt
- 1/4 teaspoon black pepper
- 4 cups vegetable broth
- 1 small onion, sliced
- 1 red tomato, chopped
- 1/4 cup parsley

Directions:
1. Heat the oil in a large saucepan or soup pot.
2. Stir in the celery, onion, and thyme.
3. Sauté approximately for 5 minutes, occasionally stirring, until the vegetables are soft.
4. Add the garlic and sauté for approximately 30 seconds until it is fragrant.
5. Stir in the zucchini, green beans, salt, and pepper.
6. Sauté for approximately 2 minutes, until these vegetables are slightly soft.
7. Add the broth and tomato.
8. Increase the temperature to high and bring the mixture to a boil.
9. Reduce the heat to low; cover the pan with the lid, and simmer for 10 minutes.
10. Chop the parsley and stir it in.
11. Remove from the heat.
12. Serve hot.

Nutrition:
- **Calories:** 371
- **Total Carbs:** 13.6 g
- **Net Carbs:** 9.9 g
- **Fat:** 31 g
- **Protein:** 13 g

17. Chili With Beef

Preparation Time: 35 minutes
Cooking Time: 6–8 hours
Servings: 2
Ingredients:
- 1/3 lb. ground beef
- 2/3 cans diced tomatoes with green chilies
- 2/3 white onions, diced
- 1 1/3 garlic cloves, minced
- 1/2 tablespoon Mexican seasoning
- 2 oz. tomato paste
- A pinch of salt and ground black pepper
- Cilantro (optional, for serving)
- Grated cheese (optional, for serving)
- Sour cream (optional, for serving)

Directions:
1. Place a large skillet pan over medium-high heat, add the beef, half of both garlic and onion, and a pinch of salt and ground black pepper.
2. Cook for 5 to 7 minutes, stirring regularly until the meat is nicely golden brown.
3. Drain off the fat and add to the slow-cooker.
4. Stir in the remaining ingredients and place the lid on the slow-cooker.
5. Set the cooking timer for 6 to 8 hours and cook at a low heat setting.
6. To serve, allow people to help themselves to cilantro, grated cheese, and sour cream.

Nutrition:
- **Calories:** 306
- **Carbs:** 13 g
- **Net Carbs:** 10 g
- **Fat:** 18 g
- **Protein:** 23 g

18. Low Carb Chicken

Preparation Time: 15 minutes
Cooking Time: 20 minutes
Servings: 3
Ingredients:
- 3 tablespoons olive oil
- Salt and black pepper to taste
- Water, as needed
- 3 medium chicken breasts, boneless
- ½ cup onion, chopped
- 3 garlic cloves, minced
- 4 oz can green chilies, chopped
- ½ cup heavy cream
- 1/4 cup cheddar, jack cheese

Directions:
1. Cut the chicken into bite-size pieces; sprinkle salt and pepper to taste.
2. Heat oil in a large skillet, using medium heat.
3. Cook the chicken until it is brown on both sides; add the onions at the same time as you flip the chicken over.
4. Add garlic; cook for 1 minute.
5. If necessary, deglaze the pan with water.
6. Add in the green chilies and cream; simmer until the chicken is completely cooked, and the sauce has thickened.
7. Top with the shredded cheese; wait until the cheese melts.
8. Serve.

Nutrition:
- **Calories:** 503
- **Total Carbs:** 3 g
- **Net Carbs:** 2 g
- **Fat:** 33 g
- **Protein:** 45 g

19. Chicken Drumsticks

Preparation Time: 60 minutes
Cooking Time: 20 minutes
Servings: 3
Ingredients:
- lbs. chicken drum sticks skin on

Sauce:
- 2 tablespoons sesame oil
- 1/3 cups water
- 4 tablespoons vinegar
- 1/2 cup stevia
- 3 garlic cloves, minced
- 1 tablespoon ginger, grated
- 2 teaspoons red pepper flakes

Directions:
1. Combine all the sauce ingredients in a large bowl.
2. Put the chicken and sauce in a Ziploc® freezer bag; put in the freezer until the chicken is completely frozen.
3. Put chicken and sauce in the Instant Pot.
4. Close the lid and lock it.
5. Set the vent to Sealing.
6. Cook on high pressure for 15 minutes.
7. When the timer beeps, naturally release the steam for 10–15 minutes.
8. Open the lid.
9. Meanwhile, line a baking sheet with parchment paper and turn on the oven broiler.
10. Transfer the drumsticks from the Instant Pot to the baking sheet.
11. Brush the chicken with the sauce from the Instant Pot.
12. Place the chicken under the broiler for 5 minutes on each side.
13. Remove to a serving platter.
14. Serve.

Nutrition:
- **Calories:** 130
- **Total Carbs:** 2 g
- **Net Carbs:** 6 g
- **Fat:** 9 g
- **Protein:** 0.5 g

20. Chicken Curry

Preparation Time: 10 minutes
Cooking Time: 20 minutes
Servings: 4
Ingredients:
- 2 lbs. chicken, chopped
- 4 tablespoons olive oil
- 4 green pepper small, chopped
- 3 inches ginger, chopped
- 2 garlic cloves, chopped
- 4 onions, finely chopped
- 4 tomatoes, finely chopped
- 1 cup water
- 1 tablespoon lemon juice
- ½ cup fresh cilantro to garnish

Whole Spices:
- 2 black cardamoms
- 2 bay leaves
- 4 cloves
- 2 pinches black pepper
- 1/3 teaspoon cumin seeds
- 2 teaspoons coriander powder
- 1/2 tablespoons cayenne
- Salt, to taste

Directions:
1. Warm the oil in the Instant Pot, using the sauté mode.
2. Now add in the whole spices; cook for 20 seconds.
3. Stir in the onions, green chili, ginger, and garlic; cook for approximately 5 minutes (until they turn golden brown.)
4. Add the tomatoes and cook for another 4 minutes.
5. Stir in the chicken; cook for 2–4 minutes. Combine the water with the other ingredients. Deglaze; scrape off the bottom.
6. Close the lid and lock it. Set the vent to Sealing.
7. Cook on high pressure for 6 minutes.
8. When the timer beeps, quickly release the steam.
9. Open the lid. Pour in the lemon juice.
10. Remove from Instant Pot to serving platter; top with cilantro.
11. Serve.

Nutrition:
- **Calories:** 555 **Total Carbs:** 20.6 g **Net Carbs:** 15 g **Fat:** 21 g **Protein:** 69 g

21. Green Curry Shrimp and Vegetables

Preparation Time: 10 minutes
Cooking Time: 15 minutes
Servings: 4

Ingredients:
- 1 tablespoon coconut oil
- 1 small red onion, halved and sliced
- 1 eggplant, cut into 1-inch dice
- 1 head broccoli, cut into florets
- 3 tablespoons green curry paste
- 1 red bell pepper, cut into 2-inch-thick strips
- ½ pound green beans, trimmed and cut into 2-inch pieces
- 2 (14-oz.) cans coconut milk
- 2 tablespoons fish sauce
- 1 pound large shrimp, peeled
- ¼ cup coarsely chopped fresh cilantro
- 2 tablespoons freshly squeezed lime juice
- 2 or 3 drops of liquid stevia

Directions:
1. Heat a large pot over medium-high heat until hot, then pour in the oil and tilt to coat the bottom.
2. Add the onion, and cook for 2 to 3 minutes, or until beginning to soften.
3. Add the eggplant and broccoli, and cook for 2 to 3 minutes, or until beginning to soften.
4. Add the curry paste and cook for about 1 minute, or until fragrant.
5. Add bell pepper, green beans, coconut milk, and fish sauce. Bring to a simmer and cook for 5 minutes, or until the vegetables are crisp-tender.
6. Add the shrimp, cover the pot, and cook for 2 to 3 minutes, or until the shrimp are just cooked through. Do not overcook.
7. Remove from the heat and stir in the cilantro, lime juice, and stevia.

Nutrition:
- **Calories:** 704
- **Fat:** 55 g
- **Saturated Fat:** 46 g
- **Sodium:** 1905 mg
- **Total Carbs:** 34 g
- **Net Carbs:** 20 g
- **Fiber:** 14 g
- **Sugar:** 15 g
- **Protein:** 30 g

22. Mussels Veracruz

Preparation Time: 10 minutes
Cooking Time: 15 to 20 minutes
Servings: 4
Ingredients:
- 2 tablespoons extra virgin olive oil
- 1 onion, diced
- 1 tablespoon minced garlic
- 1 serrano chile, minced
- 1 (15-oz.) can whole plum tomatoes, hand crushed
- ½ cup coarsely chopped pitted green olives
- ¼ cup drained capers
- 3 fresh oregano sprigs, stemmed and minced
- 2 fresh marjoram sprigs, stemmed and minced
- 2 bay leaves
- 2 pounds fresh mussels, scrubbed and debearded
- ½ cup dry white wine

Directions:
1. Heat a large skillet over medium heat until hot, then pour in the oil and tilt to coat the bottom.
2. Add the onion, garlic, and chile, and cook for 5 minutes, or until beginning to soften.
3. Add the tomatoes, olives, capers, oregano, marjoram, and bay leaves, and cook for about 2 minutes, or until fragrant.
4. Add the mussels, then add the white wine. Cover with a tight-fitting lid and simmer for 8 to 10 minutes. All the mussels should have opened by then. Any that don't open after 10 minutes should be discarded.

Nutrition:
- **Calories:** 349
- **Fat:** 18 g
- **Saturated Fat:** 3 g
- **Sodium:** 1975 mg
- **Total Carbs:** 16 g
- **Net Carbs:** 13 g
- **Fiber:** 3 g
- **Sugar:** 4 g
- **Protein:** 21 g

23. Italian Sausage and Mussels

Preparation Time: 5 minutes
Cooking Time: 25 minutes
Servings: 4
Ingredients:
- 8 oz. hot Italian sausage, casings removed, crumbled
- 1 medium onion, finely diced
- 1 tablespoon minced garlic
- 1 cup dry red wine
- 2 tablespoons tomato paste
- 2 cups chicken stock
- 1½ pounds fresh mussels, scrubbed and debearded
- 1 cup coarsely chopped fresh basil

Directions:
1. Heat a large skillet over medium-high heat until hot.
2. Put the sausage in the skillet, and cook for 5 to 7 minutes, or until just cooked through. Transfer to a small bowl.
3. Add the onion to the skillet, and cook for 5 minutes, or until beginning to soften.
4. Add the garlic, and cook for 30 seconds, or just until fragrant.
5. Add the red wine, scraping up the browned bits from the bottom.
6. Stir in the tomato paste and chicken stock, and bring to a simmer.
7. Add the mussels, cover with a tight-fitting lid, and steam for 8 to 10 minutes. All the mussels should have opened by then. Any that don't open after 10 minutes should be discarded.
8. Stir in the basil and sausage and any accumulated juices.

Nutrition:
- **Calories:** 330
- **Fat:** 14 g
- **Saturated Fat:** 4 g
- **Sodium:** 1092 mg
- **Total Carbs:** 12 g
- **Net Carbs:** 10 g
- **Fiber:** 2 g
- **Sugar:** 3 g
- **Protein:** 26 g

24. Breaded Fish with Mustard & Basil Sauce

Preparation Time: 5 minutes
Cooking Time: 20 minutes
Servings: 4
Ingredients:
- 2 lbs. cod fillet, sliced into strips
- Salt and pepper to taste
- 16 tablespoons basil
- 3 teaspoon garlic
- 1 teaspoon dried oregano
- 8 tablespoons olive oil
- ¼ cup fresh lemon juice
- 2 teaspoon Dijon mustard

Directions:
1. Season the fish with salt and pepper.
2. Set the Instant Pot to sauté.
3. Fry each strip in olive oil until golden.
4. Set aside.
5. Add the garlic to the pot.
6. Saute for 30 seconds.
7. Add the rest of the ingredients.
8. Simmer for 2 minutes.
9. Drizzle the sauce over the fish strips before serving.

Nutrition:
- **Calories:** 152
- **Total Fat:** 4 g
- **Saturated Fat:** 3 g
- **Cholesterol:** 36 mg
- **Sodium:** 357 mg
- **Total Carbs:** 7 g
- **Dietary Fiber:** 0.5 g
- **Total Sugars:** 0.4 g
- **Protein:** 21 g
- **Potassium:** 273 mg

25. Trout and Fennel Parcels

Preparation Time: 5 minutes
Cooking Time: 20 minutes
Servings: 4
Ingredients:
- ½ lb. deboned trout, butterflied
- Salt and black pepper to season
- 3 tablespoons olive oil + extra for tossing
- 4 sprigs rosemary
- 4 sprigs thyme
- 4 butter cubes
- 1 cup thinly sliced fennel
- 1 medium red onion, sliced
- 8 lemon slices
- 3 teaspoons capers to garnish

Directions:
1. Preheat the oven to 400°F. Cut out parchment paper wide enough for each trout.
2. In a bowl, toss the fennel and onion with a little bit of olive oil and share it into the middle parts of the papers.
3. Place the fish on each veggie mound, top with a drizzle of olive oil each, a pinch of salt and black pepper, a sprig of rosemary and thyme, and 1 cube of butter.
4. Also, lay the lemon slices on the fish.
5. Wrap and close the fish packets securely, and place them on a baking sheet. Bake in the oven for 15 minutes and remove once ready.
6. Plate them and garnish the fish with capers and serve with a squash mash.

Nutrition:
- **Calories:** 234
- **Fat:** 3 g
- **Net Carbs:** 8 g
- **Protein:** 17 g

CHAPTER 4:

Dinner

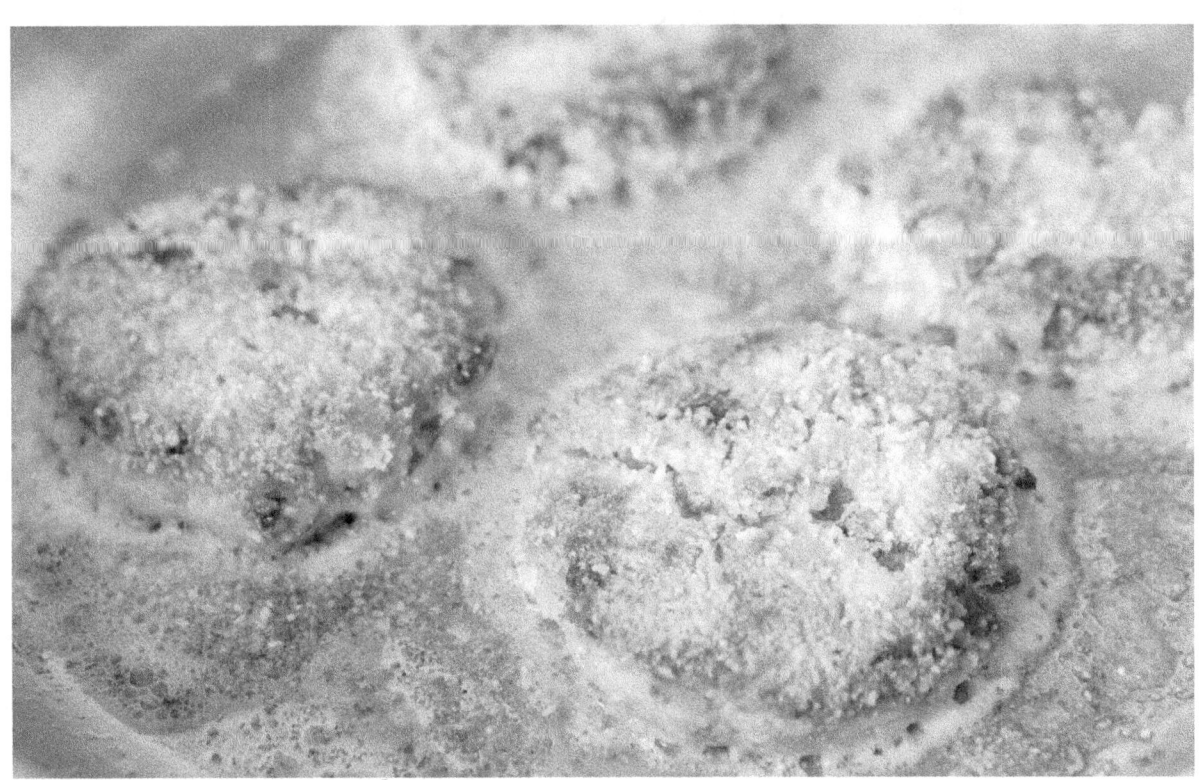

1. Salmon Panatela

Preparation Time: 5 minutes
Cooking Time: 22 minutes
Servings: 4
Ingredients:
- 1 lb. skinned salmon, cut into 4 steaks each
- 1 cucumber, peeled, seeded, cubed
- Salt and black pepper to taste
- 8 black olives, pitted and chopped
- 1 tablespoon capers, rinsed
- 2 large tomatoes, diced
- 3 tablespoons red wine vinegar
- ¼ cup thinly sliced red onion
- 3 tablespoons olive oil
- 2 slices zero carb bread, cubed
- ¼ cup thinly sliced basil leaves

Directions:
1. Preheat a grill to 350°F and prepare the salad. In a bowl, mix the cucumbers, olives, pepper, capers, tomatoes, wine vinegar, onion, olive oil, bread, and basil leaves. Let sit for the flavors to incorporate.
2. Season the salmon steaks with salt and pepper; grill them on both sides for 8 minutes in total. Serve the salmon steaks warm on a bed of the veggies salad.

Nutrition:
- **Calories:** 338
- **Fat:** 27 g
- **Net Carbs:** 1 g
- **Protein:** 25 g

2. Blackened Fish Tacos with Slaw

Preparation Time: 5 minutes
Cooking Time: 20 minutes
Servings: 4
Ingredients:
- 1 tablespoon olive oil
- 1 teaspoon chili powder
- 2 tilapia fillets
- 1 teaspoon paprika
- 4 low-carb tortillas

Slaw:
- ½ cup red cabbage, shredded
- 1 tablespoon lemon juice
- 1 teaspoon apple cider vinegar
- 1 tablespoon olive oil
- Salt and black pepper to taste

Directions:
1. Season the tilapia with chili powder and paprika. Heat the olive oil in a skillet over medium heat.
2. Add tilapia and cook until blackened, about 3 minutes per side. Cut into strips. Divide the tilapia between the tortillas. Combine all slaw ingredients in a bowl and top the fish to serve.

Nutrition:
- **Calories:** 268
- **Fat:** 20 g
- **Net Carbs:** 5 g
- **Protein:** 18 g

3. Red Cabbage Tilapia Taco Bowl

Preparation Time: 5 minutes
Cooking Time: 20 minutes
Servings: 4
Ingredients:
- 2 cups cauliflower rice
- 2 teaspoon ghee
- 4 tilapia fillets, cut into cubes
- ¼ teaspoon taco seasoning
- Salt and chili pepper to taste
- ¼ head red cabbage, shredded
- 1 ripe avocado, pitted and chopped

Directions:
1. Sprinkle cauliflower rice in a bowl with a little water and microwave for 3 minutes. Fluff after with a fork and set aside. Melt ghee in a skillet over medium heat, rub the tilapia with the taco seasoning, salt, and chili pepper, and fry until brown on all sides, for about 8 minutes in total.
2. Transfer to a plate and set aside. In 4 serving bowls, share the cauliflower rice, cabbage, fish, and avocado. Serve with chipotle lime sour cream dressing.

Nutrition:
- **Calories:** 269
- **Fat:** 24 g
- **Net Carbs:** 4 g
- **Protein:** 15 g

4. Sicilian-Style Zoodle Spaghetti

Preparation Time: 5 minutes
Cooking Time: 10 minutes
Servings: 2
Ingredients:
- 4 cups zoodles (spiraled zucchini)
- 2 oz. chopped bacon
- 4 oz. canned sardines, chopped
- ½ cup canned chopped tomatoes
- 1 teaspoon minced garlic

Directions:
1. Pour some of the sardine oil into a pan. Add garlic and cook for 1 minute. Add the bacon and cook for 2 more minutes. Stir in the tomatoes and let simmer for 5 minutes. Add zoodles and sardines and cook for 3 minutes.

Nutrition:
- **Calories:** 172
- **Fat:** 4 g
- **Fiber:** 0.6 g
- **Carbs:** 3 g
- **Protein:** 34 g

5. Sour Cream Salmon with Parmesan

Preparation Time: 5 minutes
Cooking Time: 25 minutes
Servings: 4
Ingredients:
- 1 cup sour cream
- ½ tablespoon minced dill
- ½ lemon, zested and juiced
- Pink salt and black pepper to season
- 4 salmon steaks
- ½ cup grated Parmesan cheese

Directions:
1. Preheat oven to 400°F and line a baking sheet with parchment paper; set aside. In a bowl, mix the sour cream, dill, lemon zest, juice, salt, and black pepper, and set aside.
2. Season the fish with salt and black pepper, drizzle lemon juice on both sides of the fish, and arrange them on the baking sheet. Spread the sour cream mixture on each fish and sprinkle with Parmesan.
3. Bake the fish for 15 minutes and after broil the top for 2 minutes with a close watch for a nice brown color. Plate the fish and serve with buttery green beans.

Nutrition:
- **Calories:** 355
- **Fat:** 31 g
- **Net Carbs:** 6 g
- **Protein:** 20 g

6. Roasted Tomato and Chicken Pasta

Preparation Time: 20 min
Cooking Time: 30 min
Servings: 4

Ingredients:
- 1 pound boneless, skinless chicken thighs, cut into bite-size pieces
- ⅛ teaspoon kosher salt (optional)
- ¼ teaspoon freshly ground black pepper (optional)
- 4 cups cherry tomatoes, halved
- 4 garlic cloves, minced
- 1 tablespoon canola or sunflower oil
- 1 teaspoon dried basil
- 8 oz. uncooked whole-wheat rotini
- 10 Kalamata olives, pitted and sliced
- ¼ teaspoon red pepper flakes (optional)
- ¼ cup grated Parmesan cheese (optional)

Directions:
1. Preheat the oven to 450°F.
2. Season the chicken with salt and pepper, if desired. Toss the chicken in a large bowl with tomatoes, garlic, oil, and basil. Transfer to a rimmed baking sheet and spread out evenly.
3. Roast until the chicken is cooked through 15 to 20 minutes, tossing halfway through. A meat thermometer should read 165°F.
4. Meanwhile, cook the pasta to al dente according to the package directions. Drain.
5. In a large serving bowl, toss the chicken and tomatoes with the pasta, olives, and pepper flakes (if using). Top with Parmesan, if desired.

Nutrition:
- **Calories:** 458
- **Total Fat:** 14 g
- **Saturated Fat:** 3 g
- **Cholesterol:** 110 mg
- **Sodium:** 441 mg
- **Carbs:** 52 g
- **Fiber:** 8 g
- **Protein:** 34 g

7. Oat Risotto with Mushrooms, Kale, and Chicken

Preparation Time: 30 minutes
Cooking Time: 30 minutes
Servings: 4
Ingredients:
- 4 cups reduced-sodium chicken broth
- 1 tablespoon extra virgin olive oil
- 1 small onion, finely chopped
- 1 pound sliced mushrooms
- 1 pound boneless, skinless chicken thighs, cut into bite-size pieces
- 1¼ cups quick-cooking steel-cut oats
- 1 (10-oz.) package frozen chopped kale (about 4 cups)
- ½ cup grated Parmesan cheese (optional)
- Freshly ground black pepper (optional)

Directions:
1. In a medium saucepan, bring the broth to a simmer over medium-low heat.
2. Warm the olive oil in a large, non-stick skillet over medium-high heat. Sauté the onion and mushrooms until the onion is translucent, about 5 minutes. Push the vegetables to the side and add the chicken. Let it sit untouched until it browns, about 2 minutes.
3. Add the oats. Cook for 1 minute, stirring constantly. Add ½ cup of the hot broth and stir until it is completely absorbed. Continue stirring in broth, ½ cup at a time, until it is absorbed and the oats and chicken are cooked, about 10 minutes. If you run out of broth, switch to hot water.
4. Stir in the frozen kale, and cook until it's warm. Top with Parmesan and black pepper, if you like.
5. **FLAVOR BOOST:** Garnish with minced parsley and red pepper flakes. You can also substitute ½ cup dry white wine for ½ cup of chicken broth.
6. **INGREDIENT TIP:** All varieties of oats have similar amounts of fiber, vitamins, and minerals. The main difference is in how quickly they're digested, with the steel-cut and old-fashioned/rolled oats breaking down more slowly, which is helpful for blood sugar control. The quick-cooking steel-cut oats used in this risotto are simply cut into smaller pieces, enabling you to make this dish in under 30 minutes.

Nutrition:
- **Calories:** 470 **Total Fat:** 16 g
- **Saturated Fat:** 4 g **Cholesterol:** 118 mg
- **Sodium:** 389 mg **Carbs:** 44 g
- **Fiber:** 9 g **Protein:** 40 g

8. Turkey and Tomato Sauce

Preparation Time: 10 minutes
Cooking Time: 7 hours
Servings: 2
Ingredients:
- 1 cup tomato sauce
- ½ cup chicken stock
- ½ tablespoon rosemary, chopped
- 1 pound turkey breast, skinless, boneless, and roughly cubed
- 1 teaspoon rosemary, dried
- 1 tablespoon cilantro, chopped
- A pinch of salt and black pepper

Directions:
1. In your slow cooker, mix the turkey with the sauce, stock and the other ingredients toss, put the lid on and cook on Low for 7 hours.
2. Divide everything between plates and serve.

Nutrition:
- **Calories:** 283
- **Fat:** 16 g
- **Fiber:** 2 g
- **Carbs:** 6 g
- **Protein:** 17 g

9. Tomato Chicken and Chickpeas

Preparation Time: 10 minutes
Cooking Time: 7 hours
Servings: 2
Ingredients:
- 1 tablespoon olive oil
- 1 red onion, chopped
- 1 cup canned chickpeas, drained
- 1 pound chicken breast, skinless, boneless, and cubed
- ½ cup tomato sauce
- ½ cup cherry tomatoes, halved
- ½ teaspoon rosemary, dried
- ½ teaspoon turmeric powder
- 1 cup chicken stock
- A pinch of salt and black pepper
- 1 tablespoon chives, chopped

Directions:
1. Grease the slow cooker with the oil and mix the chicken with the onion, chickpeas, and the other ingredients inside the pot.
2. Put the lid on, cook on Low for 7 hours, divide between plates and serve.

Nutrition:
- **Calories:** 291
- **Fat:** 17 g
- **Fiber:** 3 g
- **Carbs:** 7 g
- **Protein:** 16 g

10. Turkey with Leeks and Radishes

Preparation Time: 10 minutes
Cooking Time: 6 hours
Servings: 2
Ingredients:
- 1 pound turkey breast, skinless, boneless, and cubed
- 1 leek, sliced
- 1 cup radishes, sliced
- 1 red onion, chopped
- 1 tablespoon olive oil
- A pinch of salt and black pepper
- 1 cup chicken stock
- ½ teaspoon sweet paprika
- ½ teaspoon coriander, ground
- 1 tablespoon cilantro, chopped

Directions:
1. In your slow cooker, combine the turkey with the leek, radishes, onion, and the other ingredients toss, put the lid on and cook on high for 6 hours.
2. Divide everything between plates and serve.

Nutrition:
- **Calories:** 226
- **Fat:** 9 g
- **Fiber:** 1 g
- **Carbs:** 6 g
- **Protein:** 12 g

11. Low-Carb Pork Medallions

Preparation Time: 5 minutes
Cooking Time: 30 minutes
Servings: 6
Ingredients:

- 1 lb. pork tenderloin
- 3 medium shallots (chopped nice)
- ¼ cup oil

Directions:

1. Cut the meat into half-inch thick cuts.
2. Chop the shallots and place them on a plate.
3. Heat the oil in a skillet.
4. Rub the meat with the shallots on both sides. The shallots will stick to the pork if pressed solidly.
5. Place the meat with shallots into the warm oil and prepare dinner until accomplished. The shallots will get cooked until golden and they'll grant a delicious taste to the beef. Simply cook the meat until it's cooked through.
6. Serve with veggies.

Nutrition:

- **Carbs:** 18 g
- **Fat:** 37 g
- **Protein:** 33 g
- **Calories:** 535

12. Easy Mozzarella & Pesto Chicken Casserole

Preparation Time: 5 minutes
Cooking Time: 30 minutes
Servings: 4
Ingredients:
- ¼ cup pesto
- 8 oz. cream cheese softened
- ¼–½ cup heavy cream
- 8 oz. mozzarella cubed
- 2 lbs. cooked cubed chicken breasts
- 8 oz. mozzarella shredded
- Cooking spray
- Zoodles (optional, for serving)
- Spinach (optional, for serving)
- Squashed cauliflower (optional, for serving)

Directions:
1. Preheat the oven to 400°F. Spray a cooking dish with cooking spray.
2. Take the initial three ingredients and mix until smooth in a large bowl. Add the chicken and cubed mozzarella. Transfer to the goulash dish. Sprinkle the shredded mozzarella to finish everything.
3. Prepare for 25–30 minutes. Serve with zoodles, spinach, or squashed cauliflower.

Nutrition:
- **Calories:** 404
- **Fat:** 23 g
- **Net Carbs:** 8 g
- **Protein:** 31 g

13. Easy Taco Casserole Recipe
Preparation Time: 5 minutes
Cooking Time: 30 minutes
Servings: 4
Ingredients:
- 5 to 2 lbs. ground turkey or beef
- 2 tablespoons taco seasoning
- 1 cup salsa
- 16 oz. cottage cheese
- 8 oz. shredded cheddar cheese

Directions:
1. Preheat the oven to 400°F.
2. Blend the ground meat and taco seasoning in a big meal dish.
3. Prepare for 20 minutes.
4. In the meantime, combine the cottage cheese, salsa, and 1 part of the cheddar. Put aside.
5. Take off the meal dish from the oven and cautiously change the cooling fluid from the meat. Cut the meat into little pieces. A potato masher works incredibly for this. Spread the cheese and salsa mix over the meat. Sprinkle the rest of the cheddar to finish everything.
6. Return the meal to the oven and heat for an extra 15–20 minutes until the meat is cooked completely, and the cheddar is hot and bubbly.

Nutrition:
- **Calories:** 382
- **Fat:** 28 g
- **Net Carbs:** 3 g
- **Protein:** 22 g

14. Parmesan Chicken Tenders

Preparation Time: 5 minutes
Cooking Time: 20 minutes
Servings: 5
Ingredients:
- 1.5 lb. bag chicken tenderloins
- ¾ cup butter
- 1⅛ cup parmesan cheese
- ¾ teaspoon garlic powder
- Salt, to taste

Directions:
1. Soften the butter in a skillet and add the parmesan cheddar and garlic powder (and salt, if utilizing). Add the chicken to the mix and place it on a treat sheet. Cook at 325°F for 20–30 minutes (until the chicken is not pink inside and the juices run clear). Don't over-bake!
2. We have prepared this for Sunday lunch. My mother set them up for after church. In that case, we just have to put them on the oven in the "warm" setting for about 3½ hours while we are out. Worked incredibly!

Nutrition:
- **Calories:** 126
- **Fat:** 15 g
- **Net Carbs:** 0.3 g

15. Broccoli & Cheddar Keto Bread Recipe

Preparation Time: 5 minutes
Cooking Time: 30 minutes
Servings: 4
Ingredients:
- 5 eggs, beaten
- 1 cup shredded cheddar cheese
- ¾ cup fresh raw broccoli florets, chopped
- 3 ½ tablespoon coconut flour
- 2 teaspoon baking powder
- 1 teaspoon salt
- Cooking spray

Directions:
1. Preheat broiler to 350°F. Spray cooking spray on a skillet.
2. Mix all ingredients in a medium bowl. Fill the skillet with it.
3. Heat for 30–35 minutes or until puffed and brilliant. Cut and serve.
4. To reheat use a microwave or warmth in a greased griddle.

Nutrition:
- **Calories:** 80
- **Fat:** 5 g
- **Net Carbs:** 4 g
- **Protein:** 4 g

16. Bacon-Wrapped Chicken Tenders with Ranch Dip

Preparation Time: 5 minutes
Cooking Time: 45 minutes
Servings: 3
Ingredients:
- 12 chicken tenderloins (about 5 lbs.)
- 12 bacon slices

Ranch Dip:
- 1/3 cup sour cream
- 1/3 cup mayo
- 1 teaspoon garlic powder
- 1 teaspoon onion powder
- 1 teaspoon parsley
- 1 teaspoon dill
- ½ teaspoon salt

Directions:
1. Preheat the broiler to 400°F.
2. Wrap every chicken delicate firmly in a bit of bacon. Extend the bacon as you fold it over the chicken.
3. Place on a baking sheet. Prepare for 35–45 minutes until the bacon is fresh, and the chicken is completely cooked.
4. In the meantime, mix together the ingredients. Serve with the cooked chicken.

Nutrition:
- **Calories:** 473
- **Fat:** 40 g
- **Net Carbs:** 6 g
- **Protein:** 21 g

17. Farmhouse Beans & Sausage

Preparation Time: 6 minutes
Cooking Time: 10 minutes
Servings: 4
Ingredients:
- 2 cups gluten-free chicken broth
- 2 16-oz. frozen green beans
- 1 16-oz. chicken sausage, sliced
- ½ onion, diced
- 2 teaspoons Herb Amare
- Salt & pepper to taste

Directions:
1. Place all the ingredients in the Instant Pot. Place the top on and close it, ensuring the steam vent is shut.
2. Utilize the manual mode and set it at 6 minutes.
3. When cooking time is up, use the fast discharge strategy to let off the steam.

Nutrition:
- **Calories:** 252
- **Fat:** 21 g
- **Net Carbs:** 8 g
- **Protein:** 8 g

18. Chicken Al Forno & Vodka Sauce with Two Cheeses

Preparation Time: 10 minutes
Cooking Time: 25 minutes
Servings: 2
Ingredients:
- 2 pounds chicken breast (cooked and cut into chunks)
- 1 ½ cups vodka sauce jarred or homemade
- ½ cup parmesan cheese
- 16 oz. fresh mozzarella
- Fresh spinach (optional)

Directions:
1. Preheat the broiler to 400°F. Spray cooking spray on a cooking dish. Add the cooked chicken.
2. Top with vodka sauce, parmesan cheddar, and fresh mozzarella.
3. Heat until hot and bubbly. Around 25-30 minutes.
4. **Discretionary:** You can serve this over baby spinach. The warmth from the sauce shrinks the spinach.

Nutrition:
- **Calories:** 326
- **Fat:** 24 g
- **Net Carbs:** 5 g
- **Protein:** 21 g

19. Coconut Turkey

Preparation Time: 10 minutes
Cooking Time: 5 hours
Servings: 2
Ingredients:
- 1 yellow onion, chopped
- 1 tablespoon olive oil
- 1 cup coconut cream
- ½ teaspoon curry powder
- 1-pound turkey breast, skinless, boneless, and cubed
- 1 teaspoon turmeric powder
- ½ cup chicken stock
- 1 tablespoon parsley, chopped
- A pinch of salt and black pepper

Directions:
1. In your slow cooker, mix the turkey with the onion, oil, and the other ingredients except for the cream and the parsley, stir, put the lid on and cook on high for 4 hours and 30 minutes.
2. Add the remaining ingredients, toss, put the lid on again, cook on high for 30 minutes more, divide the mix between plates, and serve.

Nutrition:
- **Calories:** 283
- **Fat:** 11 g
- **Fiber:** 2 g
- **Carbs:** 8 g
- **Protein:** 15 g

20. Hot Chicken and Zucchinis

Preparation Time: 10 minutes
Cooking Time: 6 hours
Servings: 2
Ingredients:
- 1 pound chicken breasts, skinless, boneless, and cubed
- 1 zucchini, cubed
- 2 garlic cloves, minced
- 1 red chili, minced
- ½ teaspoon hot paprika
- 1 red onion, chopped
- 2 tablespoons olive oil
- A pinch of salt and black pepper
- 1 cup chicken stock
- 1 tablespoon chives, chopped

Directions:
1. In your slow cooker, mix the chicken with the zucchini, garlic, chili pepper, and the other ingredients toss, put the lid on and cook on low for 6 hours.
2. Divide everything between plates and serve.

Nutrition:
- **Calories:** 221
- **Fat:** 12 g
- **Fiber:** 2 g
- **Carbs:** 5 g
- **Protein:** 17 g

21. Chicken Bacon Ranch Casserole

Preparation Time: 25 minutes
Cooking Time: 2 hours 10 minutes
Servings: 6
Ingredients:
- 1 lb. chicken, shredded
- 1 onion, diced
- 1 head cauliflower, riced
- 10 oz. bacon
- 1 teaspoon salt
- 1 cup ranch dressing

Directions:
1. Preheat your oven to 400°F.
2. Place your bacon on a baking sheet and cook for 15 minutes in the oven.
3. As the bacon cooks, rice the cauliflower head and dice your onion. Combine the rice and onion, sprinkle with salt.
4. By now, the bacon is ready. Remove from the oven and set aside. Reduce the oven temperature to 350°F.
5. Place the chicken on a baking sheet and cook for 35 minutes.
6. In the meantime, chop the bacon and add to the cauliflower mixture.
7. Once the chicken is ready, shred it and add it to the mixture.
8. Add the dressing and stir until everything is completely coated.
9. Place back in the oven and cook for 30 minutes more at 350°F covered.
10. Uncover and continue to bake for 5 more minutes.
11. Turn your oven to broil and cook for 5 minutes until the top is crisp.
12. Serve immediately.

Nutrition:
- **Calories:** 400
- **Fat:** 22 g
- **Carbs:** 9 g
- **Proteins:** 41 g

22. Sushi Shrimp Rolls

Preparation Time: 5 minutes
Cooking Time: 10 minutes
Servings: 5
Ingredients:
- 2 cups cooked and chopped shrimp
- 1 tablespoon sriracha sauce
- ¼ cucumber, julienned
- 5 hand roll nori sheets
- ¼ cup mayonnaise
- 1 oz. sugar-free soy sauce

Directions:
Combine shrimp, mayonnaise, cucumber, and sriracha sauce in a bowl. Lay out a single nori sheet on a flat surface and spread about 1/5 of the shrimp mixture. Roll the nori sheet as desired. Repeat with the other ingredients. Serve with sugar-free soy sauce.

Nutrition:
- **Calories:** 216
- **Fat:** 10 g
- **Net Carbs:** 1 g
- **Protein:** 17 g

23. Grilled Shrimp with Chimichurri Sauce

Preparation Time: 5 minutes
Cooking Time: 55 minutes
Servings: 4
Ingredients:
- 1 pound shrimp, peeled and deveined
- 2 tablespoons olive oil
- 1 lime juice

Chimichurri:
- ½ teaspoon salt
- ¼ cup olive oil
- 2 garlic cloves
- ¼ cup red onions, chopped
- ¼ cup red wine vinegar
- ½ teaspoon pepper
- 2 cups parsley
- ¼ teaspoon red pepper flakes

Directions:
1. Process the chimichurri ingredients in a blender until smooth; set aside. Combine shrimp, olive oil, and lime juice in a bowl, and let marinate in the fridge for 30 minutes. Preheat your grill to medium. Add shrimp and cook for about 2 minutes per side. Serve shrimp drizzled with the chimichurri sauce.

Nutrition:
- **Calories:** 283
- **Fat:** 20.3 g
- **Net Carbs:** 5 g
- **Protein:** 16 g

24. Coconut Crab Patties

Preparation Time: 5 minutes
Cooking Time: 15 minutes
Servings: 8
Ingredients:
- 2 tablespoons coconut oil
- 1 tablespoon lemon juice
- 1 cup lump crabmeat
- 2 teaspoon Dijon mustard
- 1 egg, beaten
- 1 ½ tablespoon coconut flour

Directions:
1. In a bowl to the crabmeat, add all the ingredients except for the oil; mix well to combine. Make patties out of the mixture. Melt the coconut oil in a skillet over medium heat. Add the crab patties and cook for about 2-3 minutes per side.

Nutrition:
- **Calories:** 215
- **Fat:** 15 g
- **Net Carbs:** 6 g
- **Protein:** 13 g

25. Shrimp in Curry Sauce

Preparation Time: 5 minutes
Cooking Time: 15 minutes
Servings: 2

Ingredients:
- ½ oz. grated Parmesan cheese
- 1 egg, beaten
- ¼ teaspoon curry powder
- 2 teaspoons almond flour
- 12 shrimp, shelled
- 3 tablespoons coconut oil

Sauce:
- 2 tablespoons curry leaves
- 2 tablespoons butter
- ½ onion, diced
- ½ cup heavy cream
- ½ oz. cheddar cheese, shredded

Directions:
1. Combine all dry ingredients for the batter. Melt the coconut oil in a skillet over medium heat. Dip the shrimp in the egg first, and then coat with the dry mixture. Fry until golden and crispy.
2. In another skillet, melt butter. Add onion and cook for 3 minutes. Add curry leaves and cook for 30 seconds. Stir in heavy cream and cheddar and cook until thickened. Add shrimp and coat well. Serve.

Nutrition:
- **Calories:** 560
- **Fat:** 41 g
- **Net Carbs:** 3 g
- **Protein:** 24 g

26. Tilapia with Olives & Tomato Sauce

Preparation Time: 5 minutes
Cooking Time: 30 minutes
Servings: 4
Ingredients:
- 4 tilapia fillets
- 2 garlic cloves, minced
- 2 teaspoons oregano
- 14 oz. diced tomatoes
- 1 tablespoon olive oil
- ½ red onion, chopped
- 2 tablespoons parsley
- ¼ cup Kalamata olives

Directions:
1. Heat olive oil in a skillet over medium heat and cook the onion for 3 minutes. Add garlic and oregano and cook for 30 seconds. Stir in tomatoes and bring the mixture to a boil. Reduce the heat and simmer for 5 minutes. Add olives and tilapia, and cook for about 8 minutes. Serve the tilapia with tomato sauce.

Nutrition:
- **Calories:** 282
- **Fat:** 15 g
- **Net Carbs:** 6 g
- **Protein:** 23 g

CHAPTER 5:

Desserts

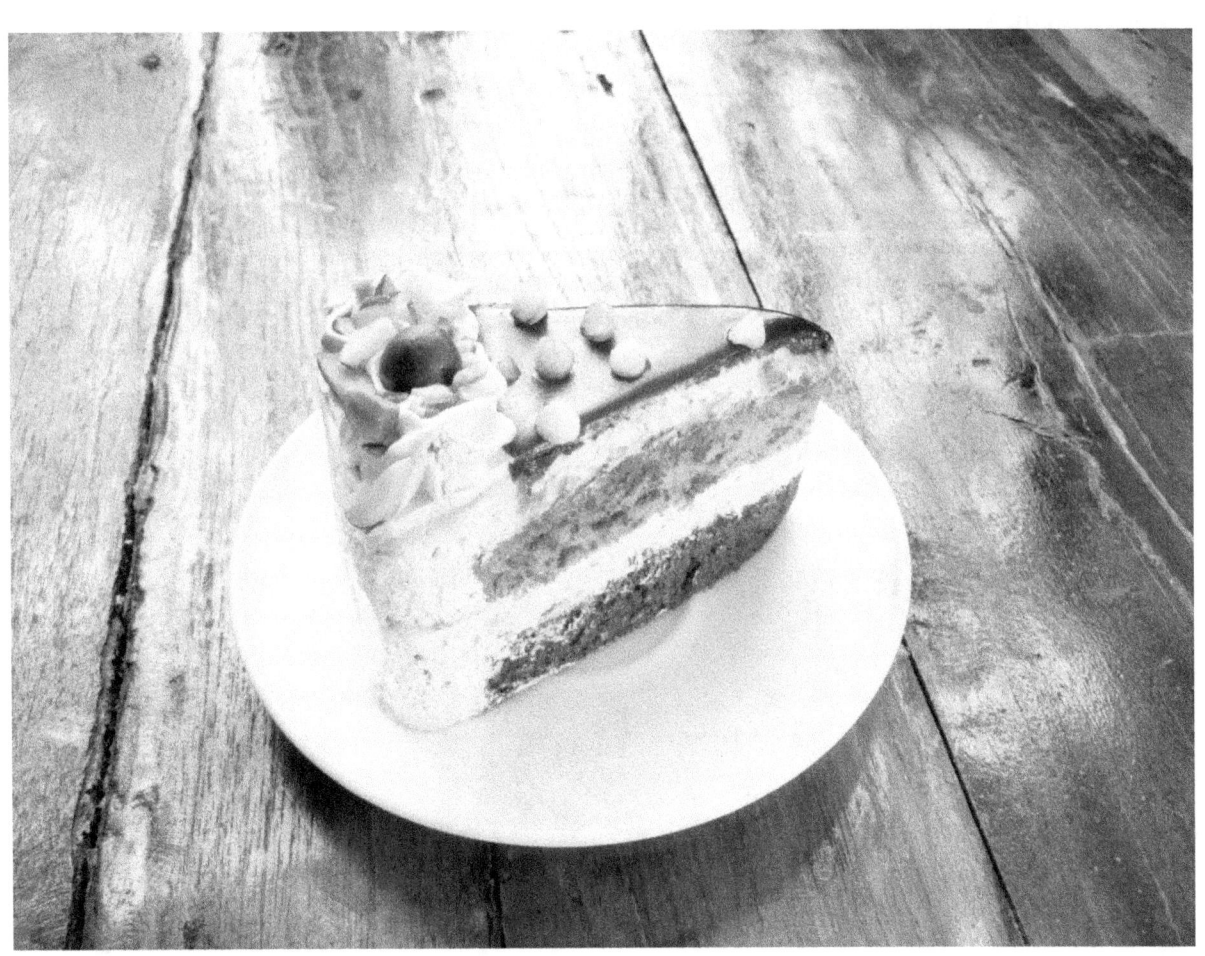

1. Berries With Chocolate Ganache

Preparation Time: 10 minutes
Cooking Time: 5 minutes
Servings: 6
Ingredients:
- 1 cup strawberries
- 2 cups raspberries
- 2 cups blueberries
- ½ cup sugar-free chocolate chips
- ⅓ cup heavy cream
- ½ teaspoon pure vanilla extract

Directions:
2. In a large bowl, combine the fruit. Stir.
3. Divide the fruit between 6 dessert bowls.
4. Boil a pot of water on medium heat. Place a glass bowl over the pot. Pour in the chocolate chips. Let melt. Stir in the cream. Remove from heat. Stir in the vanilla. Let cool slightly.
5. Pour over the fruit. Serve.

Nutrition:
- **Calories:** 260
- **Fat:** 17.8 g
- **Carbs:** 11.7 g
- **Protein:** 2.3 g
- **Dietary Fiber:** 7.4 g

2. Caramelized Pear Custard

Preparation Time: 10 minutes
Cooking Time: 20 minutes
Servings: 8
Ingredients:
- 2 tablespoons butter
- 2 tablespoons Xylitol
- ¼ teaspoon ground cardamom
- 2 medium pears
- 3 eggs
- 2 egg yolks
- 2 cups heavy cream
- 1/8 cup sugar-free low-calorie maple syrup
- ½ teaspoon rum
- 1 teaspoon pure vanilla extract

Directions:
1. Preheat the oven to 375°F.
2. Peel the pears. Slice them in half.
3. In a saucepan, over medium heat, melt the butter. Add the rum, xylitol and cardamom. Stir well.
4. Add the pears to the saucepan. Cover with sauce. Cook 4 minutes per side.
5. Transfer the pears and sauce to a deep glass dish.
6. In a small bowl, whisk the eggs, egg yolks, maple syrup, heavy cream, and vanilla until fully combined and smooth. Pour mixture over pears.
7. Bake 20 minutes, until golden brown and the custard has set.
8. Remove from oven. Cool slightly before serving.
9. Using a pastry brush, lightly brush the pears with maple syrup. Serve.

Nutrition:
- **Calories:** 310
- **Fat:** 27 g
- **Carbs:** 7.6 g
- **Protein:** 4.4 g
- **Dietary Fiber:** 1.3 g

3. Chocolate Brownie Drops

Preparation Time: 15 minutes
Cooking Time: 15 minutes
Servings: 12
Ingredients:
⅛ cup stone-ground whole wheat pastry flour
2 tablespoons whole-grain soy flour
¼ teaspoon baking powder
¼ cup unsweetened chocolate baking squares
6 tablespoons of heavy cream
2 tablespoons unsalted butter
2 large eggs
¾ cup sucralose-based sweetener

Directions:
1. Preheat the oven to 375°F.
2. Microwave the chocolate squares until almost melted. Add the butter. Stir until shiny. Set aside to cool.
3. Line a baking sheet with parchment paper.
4. In a large bowl, using an electric mixer, blend the butter until smooth. Add the sugar substitute. Blend again until smooth. Add the eggs, one at a time. Continue beating until smooth. Add the cooled chocolate to the bowl. Continue beating.
5. In a separate bowl, whisk the flour, baking powder, and soy flour.
6. Pour in the flour mixture slowly. Beat until just combined.
7. Using a rounded spoon, spoon drops of batter onto the baking sheet.
8. Bake for 5–6 minutes. Transfer to a wire rack to cool. Serve.

Nutrition:
- **Calories:** 104
- **Fat:** 9.4 g
- **Carbs:** 3.9 g
- **Protein:** 2.5 g
- **Dietary Fiber:** 3.9 g

4. Baked Pear Fans

Preparation Time: 10 minutes
Cooking Time: 40 minutes
Servings: 4
Ingredients:
- 2 medium pears
- 1 tablespoon unsalted butter
- ¼ teaspoon black pepper
- ¼ teaspoon ginger
- ¼ teaspoon cinnamon
- 1 teaspoon tap water
- ¼ teaspoon pure vanilla extract
- 1 tablespoon lemon juice

Directions:
1. Preheat the oven to 375°F.
2. You are going to make fans out of your pears. Make ¼-inch slices along the length of your half pear, starting ⅓ of an inch from the stem while cutting them all the way down to the bottom.
3. In a skillet, melt the butter. Add the lemon juice and water. Stir in the ginger, pepper, and cinnamon.
4. Place the pears in the skillet.
5. Cover with aluminum foil. Transfer skillet to the oven. Bake 40 minutes. Turn the pears halfway through cooking.
6. Using a slotted spoon, transfer pears to serving plates.
7. Place skillet on the stove. Stir in the vanilla. Simmer 1 minute.
8. Scoop the sauce over the pears. Serve.

Nutrition:
- **Calories:** 80
- **Fat:** 3 g
- **Carbs:** 11.5 g
- **Protein:** 0.4 g
- **Dietary Fiber:** 2.9 g

5. Chocolate Frosty

Preparation Time: 3 minutes
Cooking Time: 0 minutes
Servings: 1
Ingredients:
- 2 tablespoons chocolate milk
- 2 tablespoons heavy cream
- 2 tablespoons sugar-free chocolate syrup
- ½ cup ice cubes

Directions:
1. In a blender, combine the heavy cream, chocolate syrup, ice cubes. Blend until thick and smooth. Add a bit of chocolate milk for a less thick consistency. Add more ice for a thicker consistency.
2. You could chill it for 20 minutes.

Nutrition:
- **Calories:** 119
- **Fat:** 11.1 g
- **Carbs:** 0.8 g
- **Protein:** 1.6 g
- **Dietary Fiber:** 1 g

6. Ginger Flan

Preparation Time: 180 minutes
Cooking Time: 25 minutes
Servings: 6
Ingredients:
- 3 egg yolks
- 2 eggs
- 1½ cups heavy cream
- 1 cup tap water
- 8 packets sucralose-based sweetener
- 1 teaspoon pure vanilla extract
- 3 teaspoons ground ginger

Directions:
1. Preheat the oven to 350°F.
2. Place a roasting pan on the center shelf of the oven. Fill to half with boiling water.
3. In a blender, combine the eggs, egg yolks, water, cream, sugar substitute, ginger, and vanilla. Blend until smooth.
4. Pass the sauce through a sieve. Pour into a 1-quart shallow baking dish.
5. Place the dish in the water bath in the oven. Bake 30–35 minutes.
6. Transfer to a cooling rack.
7. Once cooled, spray plastic wrap with non-stick cooking spray. Place it gently against the flan. Chill in the fridge for 3 hours.
8. Once chilled, invert the baking dish and tap the flan onto a serving platter.

Nutrition:
- **Calories:** 265
- **Fat:** 26 g
- **Carbs:** 3.9 g
- **Protein:** 4.6 g
- **Dietary Fiber:** 0 g

7. Vegan Atkins Carrot Cake Bites

Preparation Time: 10 minutes
Cooking Time: 15 minutes
Servings: 6

Ingredients:
- ½ cup coconut flour
- ½ cup + 1 tablespoon water
- 2 tablespoons unsweetened applesauce
- ½ teaspoon vanilla extract
- 1 teaspoon cinnamon
- 4 tablespoons granulated monk fruit sweetener
- 1 shredded medium carrot
- 4 tablespoons unsweetened shredded coconut

Directions:
1. Mix the coconut flour, applesauce, water, and vanilla extract in a bowl and stir, blending well.
2. Now add the monk fruit sweetener, cinnamon, and shredded carrot to your mixture. Blend well.
3. Refrigerate your batter for few minutes.
4. In a separate dish, place your shredded coconut.
5. Remove the dough from the refrigerator and roll portions of it into 15 equally sized balls. Now roll the balls in the shredded coconut, coating evenly.
6. Keep refrigerated until serving.

Nutrition:
- **Calories:** 328
- **Fat:** 22 g
- **Protein:** 28 g
- **Carbs:** 8 g
- **Fiber:** 0.9 g

8. Antipasto Skewers

Preparation Time: 3 minutes
Cooking Time: 6 minutes
Servings: 12
Ingredients:
- 12 Kalamata olives, pitted
- 12 mozzarella cheese balls
- 12 small thick slices of salami
- 12 pimento-stuffed green olives
- 12 halves of jarred cherry peppers (6 peppers, cut in half)
- 12 small pepperoncini peppers

Directions:
1. Use 12 7-inch skewers. Stick one of each component on each skewer in any order of your choosing.
2. Store skewers in the refrigerator until ready to serve. These can be stored for up to a day.
3. Serve and enjoy!

Nutrition:
- **Calories:** 55
- **Fat:** 4 g
- **Carbs:** 1 g
- **Protein:** 2 g

9. Chocolate Avocado Ice Cream

Preparation Time: 12 hours and 10 minutes
Cooking Time: 0 minutes
Servings: 6
Ingredients:
- 2 large organic avocados, pitted
- ½ cup erythritol, powdered
- ½ cup cocoa powder, organic and unsweetened
- 25 drops liquid stevia
- 2 teaspoons vanilla extract, unsweetened
- 1 cup coconut milk, full-fat and unsweetened
- ½ cup heavy whipping cream, full-fat
- 6 squares chocolate, unsweetened and chopped

Directions:
1. Scoop out the flesh from each avocado, place it in a bowl and add vanilla, milk, and cream and blend using an immersion blender until smooth and creamy.
2. Add remaining ingredients except for chocolate and mix until well combined and smooth.
3. Fold in chopped chocolate and let the mixture chill in the refrigerator for 8 to 12 hours or until cooled.
4. When ready to serve, let ice cream stand for 30 minutes at room temperature, then process it using an ice cream machine as per manufacturer instruction.
5. Serve immediately.

Nutrition:
- **Calories:** 217
- **Fat:** 14 g
- **Protein:** 8 g
- **Net Carbs:** 7 g
- **Fiber:** 4 g

10. Mocha Mousse

Preparation Time: 2 hours and 35 minutes
Cooking Time: 0 minutes
Servings: 4
Ingredients:
For the Cream Cheese:
- 8 oz. cream cheese, softened and full-fat
- 3 tablespoons sour cream, full-fat
- 2 tablespoons butter, softened
- 1 ½ teaspoon vanilla extract, unsweetened
- 1/3 cup erythritol
- ¼ cup cocoa powder, unsweetened
- 3 teaspoons instant coffee powder

For the Whipped Cream:
- 2/3 cup heavy whipping cream, full-fat
- 1 ½ teaspoon erythritol
- ½ teaspoon vanilla extract, unsweetened

Directions:
1. **Prepare cream cheese mixture:** For this, place cream cheese in a bowl, add sour cream and butter, then beat until smooth.
2. Now add erythritol, cocoa powder, coffee, and vanilla and blend until incorporated, set aside until required.
3. **Prepare whipping cream:** For this, place whipping cream in a bowl and beat until soft peaks form.
4. Beat in vanilla and erythritol until stiff peaks form, then add 1/3 of the mixture into cream cheese mixture and fold until just mixed.
5. Then add the remaining whipping cream mixture and fold until evenly incorporated.
6. Spoon the mousse into a freezer-proof bowl and place in the refrigerator for 2 ½ hours until set.
7. Serve straight away.

Nutrition:
- **Calories:** 427
- **Fat:** 42 g
- **Protein:** 6 g
- **Net Carbs:** 5 g
- **Fiber:** 2 g

11. Strawberry Rhubarb Custard

Preparation Time: 4 hours and 5 minutes
Cooking Time: 5 minutes
Servings: 5
Ingredients:
- 27 oz. coconut milk, full-fat
- 2 eggs
- ¾ cup strawberries, fresh
- ½ cup rhubarb, chopped
- ¼ cup collagen, grass-fed
- 1 teaspoon vanilla extract, unsweetened
- 1/16 teaspoon stevia, liquid
- 1/16 salt
- 1 ½ tablespoon gelatin, grass-fed
- 1 cup water

Directions:
1. Place all the ingredients in a food processor except for the gelatin and water, pulse until smooth, then add gelatin and blend until smooth.
2. Divide the custard evenly between five half-pint jars and cover with their lid.
3. Switch on the instant pot, pour in water, insert trivet stand, place jars on it, and shut the instant pot with its lid in the sealed position.
4. Press the 'manual' button, press '+/-' to set the cooking time to 5 minutes, and cook at a high-pressure setting; when the pressure builds in the pot, the cooking timer will start.
5. When the instant pot buzzes, press the 'keep warm' button, do a quick pressure release and open the lid.
6. Carefully remove the jars, let them cool at room temperature for 15 minutes or more until they can be comfortably picked up.
7. Then transfer the custard jars into the refrigerator for a minimum of 4 hours and cool completely.
8. When ready to serve, shake the jars a few times to mix all the ingredients and then serve.

Nutrition:
- **Calories:** 262
- **Fat:** 24 g
- **Protein:** 5 g
- **Net Carbs:** 3 g
- **Fiber:** 3 g

12. Energy Bites with Turmeric

Preparation Time: 15 minutes
Cooking Time: 0 minutes
Servings: 18 bites
Ingredients:
- 1 cup almond butter
- 6 tablespoons plant-based protein powder
- 3/4 cup coconut flakes (unsweetened)
- 1 teaspoon coconut oil
- 2 teaspoons turmeric
- 1/2 teaspoon maple syrup

Directions:
1. In a blender, put in the butter, half of the coconut flakes, maple syrup, coconut oil, turmeric, and protein powder. Blend until mixed well.
2. Spread the dough on a baking sheet. Refrigerate for an hour to become firm.
3. Roll the dough into 18 bites. Arrange the bites on the baking sheet. Put in the fridge for 4 hours to harden.
4. Roll each bite into the remaining coconut flakes. Serve.

Nutrition:
- **Calories:** 157
- **Fat:** 6 g
- **Carbs:** 19 g
- **Protein:** 17 g

13. Ginger and Turmeric Smoothie

Preparation Time: 15 minutes
Cooking Time: 0 minutes
Servings: 1
Ingredients:
- 1 1/2 cups coconut milk (unsweetened)
- 1 cup ice
- 2 tablespoons pure honey
- 1 teaspoon coconut oil (softened)
- 1 teaspoon turmeric
- 1 teaspoon chia seeds
- 1 teaspoon ginger (peeled and chopped)

Directions:
1. In a blender, put in the ice, turmeric, coconut milk, honey, coconut oil, and ginger. Blend until smooth.
2. Put in a glass. Stir in the chia seeds. Let the chia seeds bloom before serving.

Nutrition:
- **Calories:** 217
- **Fat:** 14 g
- **Protein:** 8 g
- **Net Carbs:** 7 g
- **Fiber:** 4 g

14. Coffee Cacao Protein Bars

Preparation Time: 20 minutes
Cooking Time: 0 minutes
Servings: 12 bars
Ingredients:
- 2 cups mixed nuts
- 18 large Medjool dates (pitted)
- 1 cup egg white protein powder
- 1/4 cup cacao nibs
- 1/4 cup cacao powder
- 5 tablespoons water
- 3 tablespoons instant coffee powder

Directions:
1. Line a square pan (8"x8") with parchment paper.
2. In a food processor, put in the nuts, cacao powder, egg white
3. Protein and coffee. Process until the nuts are broken into small pieces only.
4. Put in the dates. Process to combine. Pour a tablespoon of water at a time while processing until the mixture becomes sticky.
5. Remove the S-blade of the processor. Stir in the cacao nibs into the mixture.
6. Pour into the lined square pan. Flatten the mixture evenly using a roller.
7. Put in the fridge for an hour. Slice into 16 bars. Serve.

Nutrition:
- **Calories:** 122
- **Fat:** 14 g
- **Protein:** 2 g
- **Net Carbs:** 7 g
- **Fiber:** 0 g

15. Mango Cream Pie

Preparation Time: 20 minutes
Cooking Time: 30 minutes
Servings: 4
Ingredients:
Crust:
- ½ cup rolled oats
- 1 cup cashews
- 1 cup dates, pitted

Filling:
- 2 mangos, large, peeled, and chopped
- ½ cup water
- 1 cup coconut milk, canned
- ½ cup coconut, shredded and unsweetened

Directions:
1. Get out a food processor and pulse all of your crust ingredients together. Press into an eight-inch pie pan.
2. Blend all filling ingredients. It should be thick and make sure it's smooth.
3. Pour it into the crust and smooth out. Allow it to set in the freezer for thirty minutes.
4. Allow it to come to room temperature for ten to fifteen minutes before slicing.

Nutrition:
- **Calories:** 485
- **Fat:** 37 g
- **Net Carbs:** 7 g
- **Protein:** 38 g

Conclusion

Being on a diet is hard—being on the Atkins diet requires a lot of effort from your side. The good news is that the effort is quickly followed by the results. Whenever you feel like you made a small victory, take the time to acknowledge it. It doesn't matter how big the win is—did you just successfully go through dealing with sugar craving or you just lost another pound? Bravo, you deserve an applause, even if it's from yourself!

If you're a busy person (and who isn't?) you can explore some of the low-carb convenience foods out there. You'll find that Atkins provides many delicious shakes, bars, and meals, and most of them are acceptable from Phase 1 on. Other brands may also be permissible, but you should read the labels carefully to ensure you're buying what you think you are.

Even though it goes without saying, we're going to say it anyway: cutting carbs is not the total answer to good health. Try to avoid carb-free foods that have a lot of chemicals, salts, or other ingredients that can undermine your health. That includes just about all fast food. And don't forget about exercise. This will be easier as the weight comes off, and you'll probably even begin to enjoy it!

The fourth phase is really about the rest of your life, hence why we haven't given you a meal plan for that particular phase. This part is about flexibility and learning to make healthy choices over unhealthy ones. You can be a little less strict in this phase, i.e., you don't have to plan everything out quite as strictly as you did in the first phase or the second one, but it's important not to become complacent either.

If you have any concerns about starting the Atkins Diet, remember to discuss them with your doctor before you begin. It's also important to remember that the side effects we listed are only temporary, so it's really a case of gritting your teeth and working through them, to enable you to get to the green grass beyond that point! If, however, these side effects are severe or very prolonged, discuss with your doctor before you continue.

The ball's in your court now. You have the information, the tools, and the motivation. Now is the time to set up the program that will work for you. You're just four phases, or maybe only three, from having the body, the health, and the quality of life that you dream of.

In a nutshell, if you found this book helpful, please kindly take the time to leave an honest review on Amazon. Your feedback will be greatly appreciated. Thank you and best wishes to you!

www.ingramcontent.com/pod-product-compliance
Lightning Source LLC
Chambersburg PA
CBHW081417080526
44589CB00016B/2564